**NO MORE FLAB!
NO MORE FAT!
NO MORE CELLULITE!
NO MORE BULGES!**

In their fabulous breakthrough book *Hard Bodies,* fitness experts Gladys Portugues and Joyce Vedral proved to the world that a workout program of weight training and exercise didn't make women look like men—it made them look smooth, svelte, and beautiful.

And it proved to the women of the world that they could have a perfect body— yes, a *perfect* body—firm, toned, and gorgeously shaped.

Now they show the busy women how to do it too—but do it in just two workout sessions a week. You won't look like the guys in *Pumping Iron.* You'll just look and feel ten years younger—and sexier—and absolutely great!

GLADYS PORTUGUES has appeared in *Self* and *Cosmopolitan,* and on the covers of *Ms., American Photographer, Muscle and Fitness, Shape,* and *Flex* magazines. She has been a guest on the *Phil Donahue* show and appeared in the film *Pumping Iron II.* As a participant in the Women's Olympia international competition, she took the prize for Best Improved Bodybuilder.

JOYCE VEDRAL is a regular contributor to *Muscle and Fitness* magazine, the author of *Now or Never,* the co-author of *Hard Bodies,* and the co-author with Rachel McLish of *Perfect Parts.* Joyce is also an expert on motivational techniques, and has written several books on that subject. She has been a guest on the *Oprah Winfrey* show.

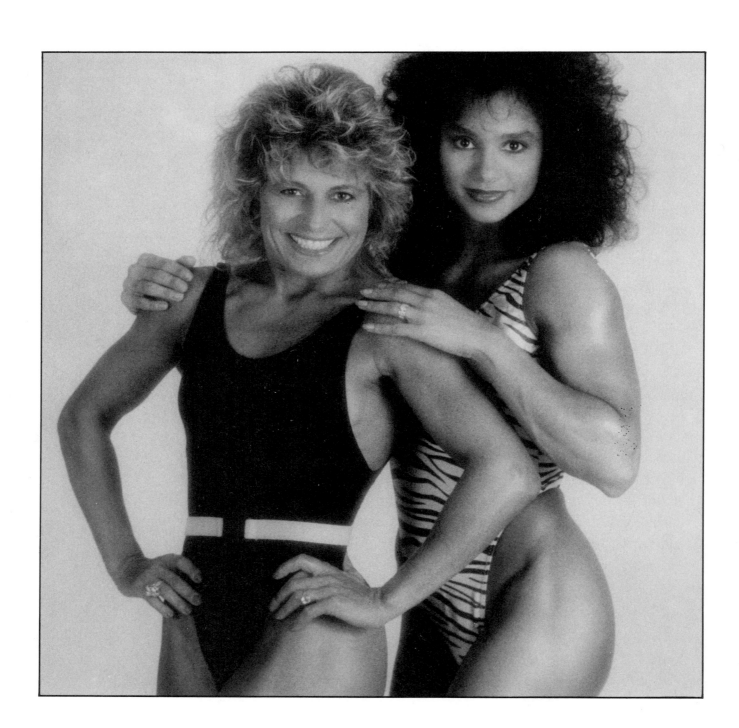

HARD BODIES
EXPRESS WORKOUT

THE TWICE-A-WEEK FITNESS PROGRAM THAT REALLY WORKS

Gladys Portugues and Joyce L. Vedral, Ph.D.

Photographs by Paul B. Goode

A DELL TRADE PAPERBACK

Published by
Dell Publishing
a division of
The Bantam Doubleday Dell Publishing Group, Inc.
1 Dag Hammarskjold Plaza
New York, New York 10017

Designed by Richard Oriolo

Dell ® TM 681510, Dell Publishing Co., Inc.

ISBN 0-440-53426-7

Printed in the United States of America

February 1988

10   9   8   7   6   5   4   3   2   1

MV

To the women who
in spite of a busy schedule
are willing to invest a few hours a week in order
to achieve and maintain
a perfectly formed, sensual body.

ACKNOWLEDGMENTS

Thank you, Joe Weider, for your expertise and continual support, and for being the first to promote feminine fitness through the vehicle of bodysculpting with weights.

Thank you, Ken Wheeler and Mohammed Makkaeay, for the fine training assistance you have offered throughout the years.

Thank you, Paul B. Goode, for your aesthetic photography, both for the cover and for the interior photographs.

Thank you, Gary Luke, editor of *Hard Bodies,* for your vision for this book.

Thank you, Marilyn Abraham, for your expertise in overseeing this project.

Thank you, Judy Davidoff, for your relentless patience in dealing with every obstacle involved with this project, and for your sensitive and alert editing of the manuscript.

Thank you, Jody Rein, for seeing this project through its final stages.

Thank you, Diane Eckablad, for being there every step of the way in the publicity efforts for this book.

Thank you, Rick Balkin, our wonderful agent, for your belief in our work and for your brilliant handling of every potential problem.

Thank you, Barbara Vale, for giving of your time in helping us to train the first women who tried this program.

Thank you, Reebok, for supplying gym shoes.

Thank you, family and friends, for your continual support.

CONTENTS

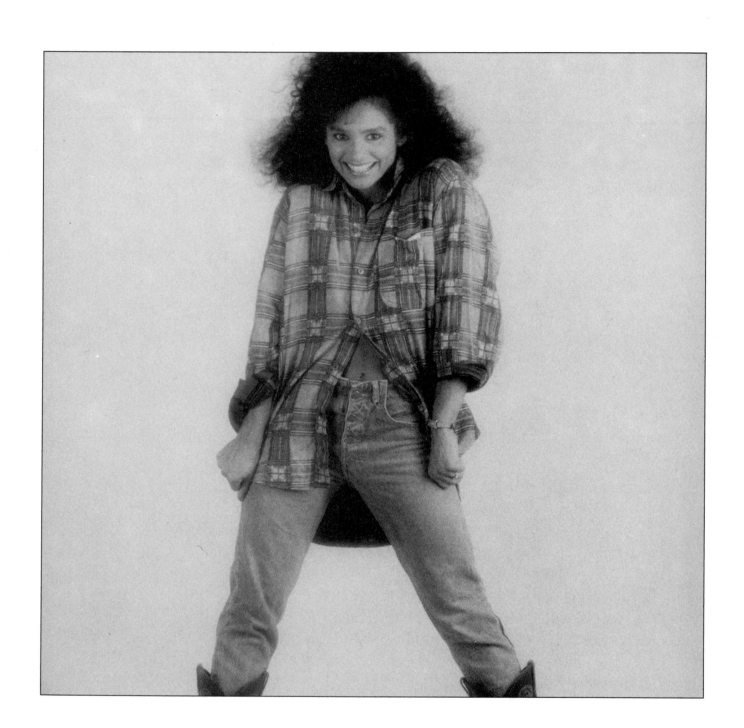

THE TWICE-A-WEEK FITNESS PROGRAM THAT REALLY WORKS

Wouldn't it be wonderful if we all had the time and the energy to work out for four or five days a week? Chances are, however, you are either too busy or too tired to invest so much time in getting into shape. Still, you desire a toned, sensual body. We invented the Hard Bodies Express Workout for you. It will get you into splendid shape with a time investment of only seventy-five minutes, two days a week.

HOW THIS PROGRAM WAS DISCOVERED

When our book *Hard Bodies* came out, we were delighted to see how many women were able to transform their bodies by following our program, which requires four workout days per week. Yet, time and time again, these same women reported to us that they had friends who expressed an interest in getting into shape but couldn't spend that much time working out. Furthermore, some women did not want to join a gym and preferred to work out at home. We decided to experiment with a revolutionary program, and to our delight, it worked. Here it is: The two-day-a-week workout—at the gym or at home—

that really achieves results. We saw dramatic changes in the women who tested out the program in a matter of months. Why does this program work?

WHY THIS PROGRAM WORKS

This program is based upon the principles stressed in *Hard Bodies*, but it is a condensed express workout. In *Hard Bodies*, the body is divided in half. Alternate parts of the body are exercised on alternate days. That is, for instance, the upper body is exercised on workout days one and three and the lower body is exercised on workout days two and four. This system is called the "split routine." In this new express workout, the entire body is exercised at each workout, thus eliminating the need for the two extra workout days. You can't work out on consecutive days, but you can work out a third day if you so desire. Three days per week is the maximum and it is extra—and not a prerequisite for getting into shape with the Hard Bodies Express Workout.

WHAT'S THE CATCH?

First, this program requires that you *never* work out two days in a row. The muscles need at least thirty-six to forty-eight hours to recuperate. It doesn't matter if you work out two days in a row when you're following a split routine, since that system provides a natural rest for the half of the body that isn't exercised on that particular day.

The other catch is that you will be doing fewer exercises than those women who work out on a split routine like the one developed in the original *Hard Bodies* workout. In the express workout, you'll only be doing two exercises a bodypart instead of four. But because of the intensity of the program, you'll still achieve a dramatically transformed body—you'll begin to see some changes in just three weeks. In three months you'll notice that your body is becoming reshaped, and in six months you will be amazed to see a total transformation of previously unsightly bodyparts.

THE GOOD NEWS FOR HARD BODIES FOLLOWERS

Those of you who have already gotten into great shape with *Hard Bodies* may find that your schedule has become too busy to work out four times a week. You can follow this program for a few months and then go right back into your *Hard Bodies* four-day-a-week program. Switching on and off from this program to the four-day program will result in your maintaining a perfectly formed and fit body.

FOR THOSE WHO NEVER EVER WANT TO WORK MORE THAN TWO DAYS A WEEK

Good news. You can get and maintain a beautiful body by using just this program.

FOR THOSE WHO MAY GET SO EXCITED THAT THEY WANT TO DO MORE

You can "graduate" to *Hard Bodies* exercises and work out four days a week. Then whenever your schedule gets busy, you can switch back to the quick two-day-a-week plan. But remember, on the two-day plan, you must not work two days in a row.

DIET IS NOT ENOUGH.

Lots of women say, "I am very strict with my diet, yet I am out of shape." You can only lose by dieting. You lose fat if you diet correctly, and you lose muscle if you diet incorrectly, but all you do is lose. And most often, you simply end up "Loose." The fat you lost leaves your skin sagging. If you lost muscle by crash dieting, your skin sags all the more. Your goal of a toned, firm body is not achieved—but the reverse, unfortunately, is! So dieting is not enough.

The only way to get into "shape" is to put shape on your body. What makes shape? Muscle—firm, tight, and well-proportioned—gives your body a sculpted look. By working with the weights exactly as prescribed here, you can actually mold your own body into shape. You will create natural sexy muscles under your skin to give you the dream body you've always imagined.

Don't worry. Your muscles won't grow too big. Not with this program. You would have to work out much longer, much harder, and perhaps take male hormones (steroids) in order to look like some of the heavily muscled women you may have seen in magazines or in bodybuilding shows. The muscles you will build by working with this program will be small and feminine.

WHY TRAINING WITH WEIGHTS THE WRONG WAY FAILS TO PRODUCE RESULTS

You may have wondered why some people spend half their lives in the gym, working with weights, yet get little or no visible results. In order to achieve a reshaped body, it is necessary to use the weights in a scientific manner. We have trained with champion bodybuilders for years and have learned the special techniques necessary to achieve maximum muscle toning and shaping for the minimum time investment. Here are the secrets.

THE SECRET OF THE PYRAMID TECHNIQUE

One of the best-kept secrets in the layman's fitness world is that of the pyramid technique. If you walk into nearly any popular health spa (a health club or gym where the average person is *not* a bodybuilder), you will find that most of the members do not pyramid the weights because they are unaware of the technique. We've asked the gym owners why they don't teach their members how to pyramid, and they tell us one of two things: "We never heard of it" or "It's too much trouble." So, for their own convenience, they keep the people working inefficiently, or out of ignorance they allow their members to spend precious time and money ineffectively.

The pyramid system has been used by champion bodybuilders since the birth of the sport and has been proven to be the best method of muscle toning, shaping, and building.

The pyramid system is not difficult to learn. You do three sets (groups of repetitions) for each exercise and you add weight to each set, *but* you do fewer repetitions for each set. Because you are doing fewer repetitions, your body is willing to try to lift the heavier weights. That's why the technique works so well.

If you were doing three sets of the side lateral raise (see p. 45), for example, and you were pyramiding your three sets, you would do fifteen repetitions for your first set at, say, five pounds. You would then pick up the next heavy weight, perhaps the eight-pound dumbbells, and you would then do ten repetitions. For your final set, you would pick up the ten-pound dumbbells and do six to eight repetitions.

Why does the pyramid system work? It appeals to the hidden psychology of your muscles. It coaxes them into growing. The first set is rather easy—a natural warm-up. The second set is a little more difficult because the weight is a bit heavier, but you realize that you don't have to do as many repetitions, so you forge ahead and manage the heavier weights. Your third set is still heavier, but you know it is your last set and that you have still fewer repetitions to do, so your body rises to the occasion and manages the last and most challenging set. Having been gently induced to work to the maximum, your muscles respond by growing firm, hard, and shapely, and they do not become overworked or injured.

The importance of the pyramid system in your workout progress cannot be overemphasized. Armed with this technique and the exercise program in chapters Four and Five, you will not have to rely on outside help that may or may not actually be helpful when it comes to assisting you to reshape your body. All you need is this book and your own determination to get into shape. That's it.

THE SECRET OF MUSCLE ISOLATION

Another best-kept secret in the layman's fitness world is that of muscle isolation. Walk into any health spa, and we have done so throughout the United States as well as in other countries, and you will see people doing exercises hit-and-miss, "as the spirit moves them," in a manner of speaking. For example, a woman will do a back exercise on the "lat pulldown" machine, and then do a chest exercise on the bench press machine, and then a triceps pushdown on the pulley pushdown. Why does she do the exercises in this order? Perhaps because the particular machines happen to be in close proximity or because a certain machine happens to be available at that moment. Perhaps because she is in the mood to do those particular exercises at that moment, perhaps because she is too tired to do the other exercises she has in mind, and so on. But such a method of exercise will *never ever* net a woman a transformed body. All that method will accomplish is the burning of a few calories and a false feeling of accomplishment.

What is muscle isolation, then? It is the working of one muscle completely before advancing to the next. For example, in this workout your chest routine requires two exercises, the bench press and the incline flye. The shoulder routine requires two exercises, the side lateral raise and the front lateral raise. In this program, you must complete your chest exercises before advancing to the shoulder exercises. You must not change the routine for the sake of convenience or mood. Only after you have finished your chest routine can you advance to your shoulder routine, and so on.

Why does muscle isolation work? It exercises the complete muscle, forcing that muscle to grow strong in order to cope with the work. When a muscle grows strong, it becomes tight, hard, and shapely. By continually skipping around and giving your muscle a rest, you destroy the concentration of effort on that muscle, and the muscle is not forced to grow.

THE SECRET OF THE MODIFIED SPLIT ROUTINE

The third best-kept secret in the nonbodybuilding fitness world is that of the split routine. The regular split routine requires that you work the upper body on workout day one and the lower body on workout day two, and so on—but with that system you must work out four days a week. The modified system operates like a split routine because instead of working two days in a row and splitting up the body, you work the entire body one day and rest completely the next day.

People who are ignorant of the split and modified split routines think, "The more the better." So they train the entire body two, three, four, five, or even seven days in a row. You would think that all this hard work would result in a greatly improved, muscular body. Ironically, the opposite sometimes is true. The muscles, instead of growing, remain the same or shrink, because muscles grow while you are at rest. Without proper rest (at least forty-eight hours), muscles cannot recuperate from the last workout. Without proper rest, your body may metabolize some of the protein in your muscle tissue in order to make up for an energy deficit, and may even shrink.

OTHER DREAMS AND FANTASIES ABOUT GETTING A PERFECT BODY

It always irks us to hear something like "I've been jogging for ten years now. Why isn't my body as beautiful as yours?" Or "For goodness' sake. I play tennis twice a week. What more do I need to look trim." Or "Well, I'm a swimmer . . ." Great. All these activities are wonderful and most help to condition your heart and lungs, and in spots they even add muscle to your body. But no activity works like correct weight training to reshape your body into perfect form. So, let's get on with the program.

ADDITIONAL BENEFITS OF WORKING WITH THIS PROGRAM

Invariably, something strange happens to women who work with this program. They become psychologically as well as physically strong. There is a mysterious carryover from the physical to the mental. For example, a woman who was previously timid may find herself standing up for her rights. Women who were always afraid of the boss feel more positive about themselves and are more inclined to act in a confident manner. These women report to us a difference in their attitude in their social and romantic lives as well. We think this psychological carryover is due to the self-esteem that comes with accomplishment, and the feeling of well-being that accompanies improved health and physical appearance.

In addition to psychological strength, one acquires discipline as a result of working with this program. "I used to give up on things when I got tired or bored," says thirty-one-year-old Lauren. "Now I plow right through it. I imagine how I will feel when the job is done. I guess it's like getting one more rep or making it through the workout and then walking out of the gym triumphantly." "This is the first thing I can say I ever really followed through on," says twenty-eight-year-old Denise. I mean I was always a quitter. Now I am using this as a base to build on."

The final and most obvious bonus is that of additional physical strength. A previously heavy load of groceries will seem light. A long, hard workday will be more tolerable. Your increased strength will show up in greater ability in your sport. You will suddenly find yourself able to open difficult doors or stuck jars, and when you go to the beach, you may be surprised to find that the beach chair and cooler are not that heavy after all.

WHAT DO YOU NEED TO GET STARTED?

All you need is this book and a gym. Or you can simply purchase minimum equipment and work out at home. It doesn't take more than three weeks to get used to the workout. At that time you'll look back and think, "It all seemed so complicated then." In a couple of months you'll go on automatic. Working out will become second nature to you. Eventually it will become as much a part of your nonnegotiable routine as brushing your teeth or taking a shower.

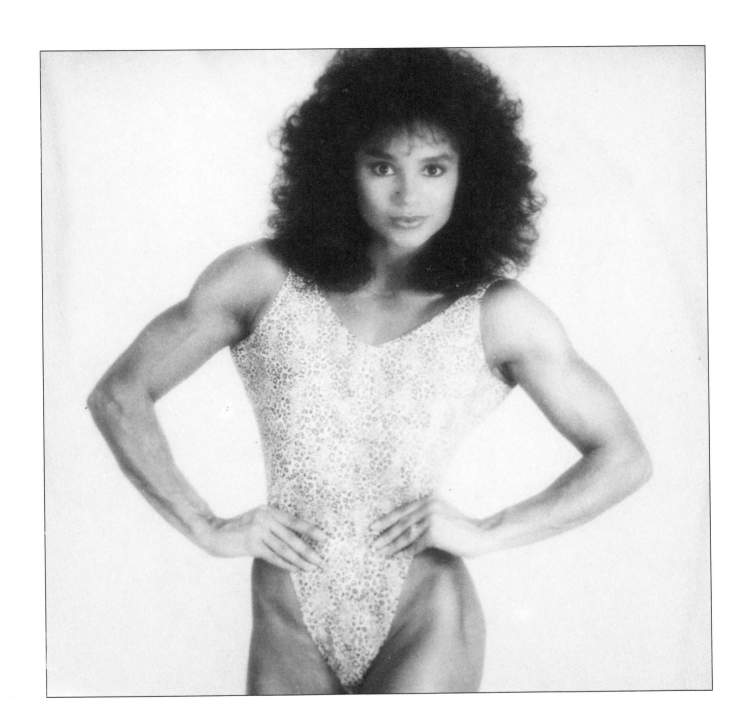

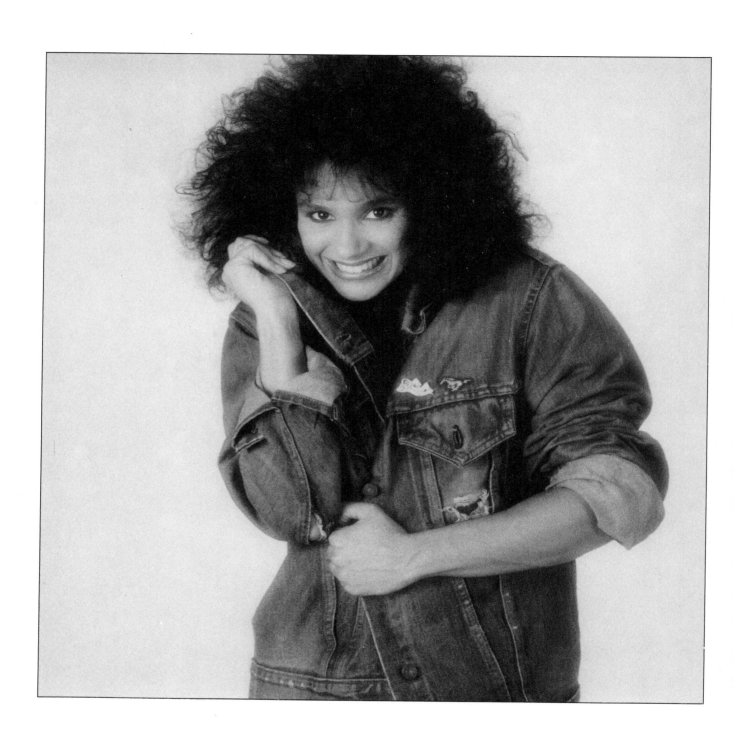

TWO

FOR BUSY AND IMPATIENT WOMEN ONLY

You're not only very busy, but you might just be about out of patience when it comes to getting into shape. You want results, and you want them "yesterday," but you have limited time to invest.

HOW MUCH TIME WILL YOU HAVE TO SPEND ON THIS PROGRAM?

You will need exactly seventy-five minutes, twice a week. That's it. If you are the ambitious type, we will allow you to do one extra workout per week, but no more than that. Anything more, with this program, would be overtraining.

HOW CAN YOU FIT THE TWO SESSIONS INTO YOUR BUSY WEEK?

Analyze your albeit full schedule and pick any two time-slots that will allow you seventy-five minutes of workout time. As noted, you can work either at home or in the gym.

When choosing your days, be sure to select days that allow at least one rest day in between. Because of the intensity of the program it is absolutely necessary to have a forty-eight-hour rest between workouts so that the muscles can recuperate and develop properly. The only muscles that do not need a rest are abdominals and buttocks. In order to become tighter and more refined, these muscles need additional stimulation to shed the excess fat that covers them.

Select a day that begins your week—Sunday, for example. Then be sure that you work out two days between Sunday and Saturday. You may choose Monday and Thursday, or Sunday and Wednesday, or Tuesday and Friday. It really doesn't matter, as long as there is at least one day of rest between workouts. You don't even have to choose the same days of each week. The idea is to get an average of two workouts in a week.

WHAT IF YOU WANT TO WORK OUT AN EXTRA DAY?

You can work out an extra day to speed your progress when you have the extra time, but be sure that you follow the rule and leave a day of rest between workouts. For example, you could work out on Monday, Wednesday, and Friday or Tuesday, Thursday, and Saturday.

WHAT IF YOU HAVE THE TIME AND YOU FEEL LIKE EXERCISING BUT YOU JUST WORKED OUT YESTERDAY?

Suppose you worked out with the program the day before but find yourself in an energetic mood today. You can work your buttocks and abdominals and, in addition, do a twenty- to thirty-minute aerobics session (jump rope, ride the stationary bicycle, run, swim, etc.). This will take you about an hour to do and you will not have overtrained. You will have burned some extra calories and worked on your buttocks and abdominals. But don't forget. Just because you put in an extra "buttocks, abdominal aerobics day" does not mean you can skip your second weekly required workout with weights. The two-day, full-seventy-five-minute weight-training sessions are a must if you want the results we guarantee.

WHY DOES THIS PROGRAM WORK FOR ALL BODY TYPES?

No matter what shape you're in, your goal is to remove unattractive, spongy fat and to replace it with firm, shapely muscles. Where will the muscles be developed and from where will the fat be removed? Muscle will be placed in each of the eight areas you exercise, and fat will be removed from your entire body, especially from areas where it tends to accumulate, such as the abdominals and the buttocks.

If you are extremely fat now, it will take you a little longer than it would a thinner person, but you will eventually achieve a hard, sensual body in six months to a year. Those of you who are thin but out of shape will take a little less time to get in shape—about four to six months. Women who are in between, and look fine in clothing but are out of shape and have too much fat on their bodies, will get to their goal between three and six months. No matter what your body looks like now, the basic principle of muscle building and fat burning will work to eventually get your body into perfect form.

HOW MUSCLES GROW

Muscles grow in response to demand. When you lift a five-pound dumbbell with each arm to do a shoulder exercise, your shoulders are put on alert. They say, "Hey, this hurts. I don't want to do this." But then, in order to cope with the task, the muscles tighten (flex), gather their forces, and do the work you demand of them. Forced into working in spite of themselves, your shoulder muscles work again when you ask them to do just a little bit more work for the next set, and so on. Your shoulder muscles (deltoids—very weak muscles on most women who have never trained with weights) will eventually become stronger and stronger, and in three months' time you will find that you can easily handle heavier dumbbells for each set of repetitions.

Muscles grow because they are not given a choice. They get tighter and stronger and denser because the muscle cells and fibers increase in size and mass in response to the added work being demanded of them. This growth process is called "muscle hypertrophy." You can see the principle of muscle hypertrophy by observing construction workers. Why are certain parts of their bodies overly developed? Their bodies have gotten stronger and thicker in response to the work demanded of them. (Don't worry, ladies. You will not build the bulk of a construction worker. They don't plan their work. Your "work" is strategically designed to produce sexy, refined, strategically-placed muscles.)

HOW FAT IS BURNED

When you perform a specific exercise, you simultaneously build hard and tight muscles while burning spongy, ugly fat—right in the area of your working muscle. In addition, each time you eat fewer calories than you expend you burn fat all over your body. This will be discussed further in Chapter Seven on eating strategies.

HOW DO YOU KNOW YOU ARE LOSING FAT?

The best way to measure fat loss is to look in the mirror. If you see firm, tight, shapely muscles where there used to be fat, you know your body composition is changing. Another way to gauge your fat loss is to feel the changing tone of your body. Poke your finger into your flexed quadriceps (thigh) area once a month and note the increasing hardness each month.

WHAT THE SCALE WEIGHS

The scale tells you what your body weight is. That includes water, muscle, fat, bone, and the like. The scale can fool you into believing that you are losing "fat" when in reality you are getting fatter. For example, you may have eaten a piece of strawberry shortcake after a huge steak dinner and you're feeling guilty. You take a double laxative and a water pill, go to bed, get up to eliminate all night long, and wake up feeling "thin" in the morning. You weigh yourself and are quite proud to see an actual loss of three pounds instead of the dreaded gain of a pound. But you have fooled yourself. What you did was to eliminate water and immediate bulk from your system. The extra calories you consumed are being stored as fat and will show up in a few days (five to seven) as a half a pound of fat on your body.

LEARNING TO USE THE MIRROR

Forget the scale. It can fool and depress you. What you see in the mirror is real. That's going to be your new scale. In other words, we want you to "sight weigh" yourself.

One final word on muscle and fat. Muscle weighs more than fat, but it takes up much less space. That is why a muscular 125-pound woman looks much slimmer than a woman weighing 120 pounds who has little muscle. Think of fat as a sponge and muscle as lead. Which takes up more space—yet which is lighter? Why should you be concerned with scale measurements? It's what you see in the mirror that counts. It's the way your clothes fit you, the way your buttocks looks in those jeans, and so on, that counts.

HOW LONG WILL IT BE BEFORE YOU SEE PROGRESS?

In two weeks you will feel as if your body has changed. You'll look in the mirror and think, "Why don't I look better yet. I feel so much tighter?" But in a month you will see a definite difference.

ONE MONTH

You will notice a clear development in your biceps muscle. That's good because it's easy to show off that muscle—you know, it's the one you use when you "make a muscle." You can have fun surprising a lot of people. You will also notice your shoulder muscles beginning to develop—a fine line here, a slight shaping there. Your pectoral muscles will begin to take form. These muscles, located under your breast area, will begin to give your breasts a firm, uplifted look. You may notice a fine line of "cleavage" developing. If you are overly "busty" you will be delighted to see that your breasts seem firmer and higher. If you are nearly flat-chested, you will be surprised to see that the firm muscles and cleavage seem to make you appear to have larger breasts.

TWO MONTHS

You will continue to see development in your biceps, shoulders, and chest, but now you will notice something happening in your triceps area. The triceps (see p. 26, anatomy photo) are the muscles that sag and wave on women who do not work out and who are not sixteen anymore. You will also notice that your trapezius muscles are beginning to form. These are located between your shoulder and neck area. You'll find that your posture is changing. You are beginning to walk with an athletic stride. This is due to the development of the latissimus dorsi muscles located in your back. They help to keep your shoulders back. The trapezius "traps" hold your head up. So the combination of the two gives you a more energetic walk.

THREE MONTHS

Now, unless you are still more than ten pounds overweight, you will see to your amazement that your abdominal (stomach) muscles are beginning to tighten. A trace of definition will be evident. You will also notice a change in your front thigh muscles (quadriceps)—a slight line of definition forming. You will see a definite change in your buttocks. They will be lifted higher and will be tighter. Dimples and "cellulite" will be reduced significantly.

SIX MONTHS

All muscles will have continued to develop, but now you'll notice a widening in your latissimus dorsi, or "lats." In addition to walking more athletically, you will *look* more like an athlete because your lats will produce a "V" look, making your waist appear smaller. Your buttocks and back thighs will have tightened and become muscular instead of spongy, and your front thigh muscles will have become still firmer and more defined.

ONE YEAR

You will be surprised to see that you have made still more progress. Even though it seemed at six months that you were nearly perfect, you will now notice that you are even tighter, shapelier, and more finely sculpted. Your abdominal area will have made much progress and now you will see small, pretty muscles there when you flex your "abs." Your buttocks will have lifted still higher and you will at last be as proud of your body in the nude as you are of it clothed.

WHY BUSY AND IMPATIENT WOMEN WILL NEVER QUIT THIS PROGRAM

"Give this up?" says Jackie, a thirty-three-year-old art director. "Not on your life. It gave me everything I dreamed about. I never thought I had the time, but then I said, oh, what the hell, it's only twice a week, and somehow I scheduled it in. When I started to see the results I got so excited that the workouts didn't seem like work at all anymore. And look at me. I'm firm and tight, and I have definition. I'm big-breasted and my breasts had no real shape. Now they're well formed and I have cleavage. I'm happy with myself for the first time in years. No way would I give this up!"

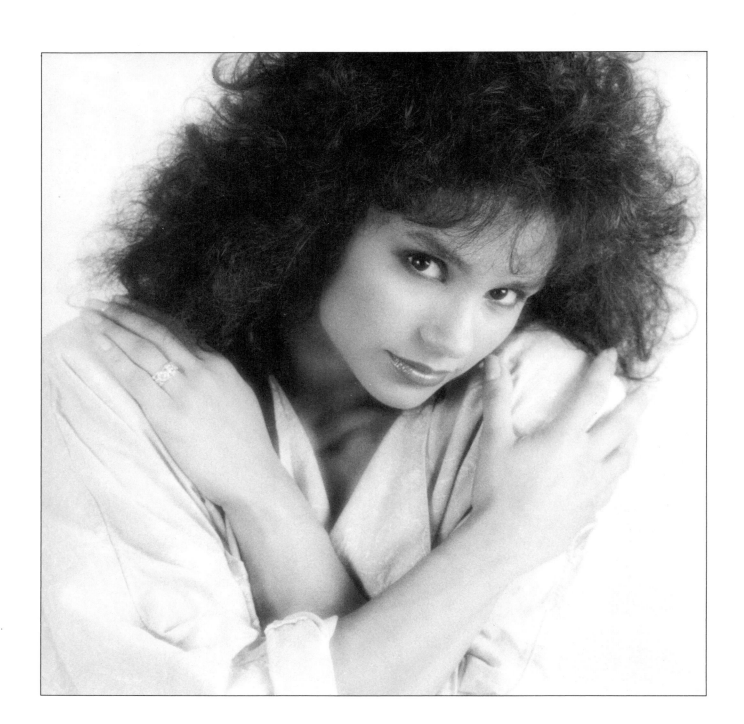

GETTING DOWN TO BUSINESS

Before you start your actual workout, there are certain things you should be aware of. How much soreness is to be expected? How long will it be before you are doing the full workout? Should you work alone or with a training partner? Are you familiar with the basic language of working out—what are a "set," a "rep," a "routine"? What's the difference between a barbell and a dumbbell? And so on.

You should also be aware of the particular muscles that will be used in the workout, so that as you exercise you can mentally concentrate on the working muscle. This chapter will describe fully your basic bodyparts: biceps, triceps, chest (pectorals), shoulder (deltoids), back (latissimus dorsi, trapezius), stomach (abdominals), buttocks (gluteus maximus), thighs (quadriceps), and so on.

Finally, in this chapter you will learn exactly how the program works. You'll discover how to select your weights, how to "pyramid," how to know when to increase your weights, and how or to what extent you can change the order of the workout described in chapters Four and Five.

Read carefully, because this is the chapter that will tell you exactly how to proceed.

MUSCLE SORENESS

When you use muscles you have never used before or have not used in a long time, you can expect a healthy amount of soreness the next day. The soreness is caused by microscopic "tears" in the connecting tissues and in the muscles themselves. These tears are not at all harmful. In fact, they are a prerequisite for muscle growth, toning, and development. Rather than dread the soreness, welcome it. It is a sign that you are making progress. In fact, if you feel no soreness after your first workout, be suspicious. Something is wrong.

Although you'll experience some soreness, the easy-does-it-break-in method allows you gradually to get used to working out. You will do one set of each exercise during your first workout, *two* sets the second workout, and three sets the third session. So in one and a half weeks, you will be completing a full workout. You will be quite sore, but still able to walk. Don't worry. You're waking your sleeping muscles from a period of hibernation, so welcome the soreness as a sign of rebirth.

HOW DO YOU KNOW THAT YOU ARE SORE AND NOT INJURED?

If you are injured, chances are, you'll *know* it. Injuries cause severe pain and are accompanied by swelling and often discoloration. If these symptoms occur, consult your doctor without delay. If, however, you are very sore, you may just *feel* as if you can hardly move. But you must not use soreness as an excuse to skip a workout.

WORK THROUGH THE SORENESS

Never, ever miss a workout because you are "too sore." The worst thing you can do is to try and wait until the soreness goes away. Kathy, a thirty-two-year-old executive editor says, "I could not walk up the stairs after my first workout. The next workout day I was so sore that I thought, This is crazy. I'll only make it worse if I go to the gym. But on faith I went and forced myself to do each exercise. Sure enough, by the time I left I felt much better. My legs were no longer stiff and cramped. I could walk down the stairs easier than before and my back felt relaxed—I could bend over again. I left the gym smiling and joking. I thought, Who would believe this? It was just as if the workout had served to massage my sore muscles."

Before I go into the specifics for starting the program, you need to acquaint yourself with a few basic bodybuilding terms.

SIMPLE BODYBUILDING TERMS

Exercise. The bodybuilding movement being executed. For example, the bench press is an exercise

Repetition (rep). One full movement of the exercise, from start point, to midpoint, to start point. For example, in the bench press exercise, the up position is start. The down position is midpoint, and the up position is back to start—the completion of one full repetition or rep.

SET. A specific number of repetitions. In this program, you will do fifteen repetitions for your first set, ten repetitions for your second set, and six repetitions for your third set. Three full sets constitute a complete exercise in this program.

PYRAMID SYSTEM. The addition of weight with the simultaneous reduction of repetitions for each set. For example, in the bench press your first set may be fifteen repetitions at twenty-five pounds. Your second set may be ten repetitions at thirty-five pounds, and your third set may be six repetitions at forty-five pounds. It is necessary to add weight to each set in order to challenge the muscle to the maximum.

REST. The pause between sets (from fifteen to forty-five seconds) so that the muscles can recuperate and gain strength for the next set.

ROUTINE. The prescribed exercises for a given bodypart. For example, in this program your chest routine consists of the bench press and the incline flye.

WORKOUT. Your entire bodybuilding program is your workout.

PROGRESSION. The gradual and continual addition of weight to the overall workout as the previous weights become too easy to lift. It is necessary to "progress" to higher weights in order to challenge the muscles to work. Unless the muscles work, they will not grow and take shape.

WORKOUT EQUIPMENT

FLAT EXERCISE BENCH. A standard gym bench used to do exercises such as the bench press or flat-bench flyes.

INCLINE BENCH. A gym bench raised to an incline (up to 45 percent) so that "incline" exercises, such as the incline bench press, incline flyes, and so on, can be performed.

DECLINE BENCH. A gym bench that is lowered to a decline so that "decline" exercises, such as the decline dumbbell press, can be performed.

BARBELL. A long bar of about three feet, which holds various evenly placed weights at either end.

DUMBBELL. A short bar of about eight inches, which can be held in each hand. Dumbbells usually have a metal ball or disc on each end.

PLATES. Disc-shaped weights used to add weight to either end of a barbell.

FREE WEIGHTS. Weights such as dumbbells and barbells, that, in contrast to weight machines, are hand-held and require the individual to do all of the work.

MACHINES. Any piece of gym equipment that is mounted to the floor and that can be used to perform a given exercise. Some of the manufacturers are Nautilus, Universal, Cybex, Paragon, David, and Kaiser. These machines afford variety and provide an extra dimension of safety, but they are not quite as effective as free weights, and should be kept to one-third or less of the workout. Only one or two exercises can be performed on each machine.

THE EASY-DOES-IT BREAK-IN METHOD

Now that you know the lingo, we can get to the program. The best way to break into this program is slowly—over a week-and-a-half period or in three workouts. Here's how.

FIRST WORKOUT DAY

On your first workout day, do only one set for each exercise. You will be doing fifteen repetitions for that first and only set that day. Your workout will take you about half an hour. (It would take less, but you are learning where the weights and machines are and you are learning how to do the exercises in strict form. It may take you forty-five minutes to an hour if you really take your time and concentrate.)

SECOND WORKOUT DAY

On your second workout day, which will be the second day of your first week, you will do two sets of each exercise. You will do your first set with fifteen repetitions, just as you did for your first workout, and then you will do another set with the heavier weight at ten repetitions. Now your workout will take about forty-five minutes because you are doing more work but are still getting used to the machines, dumbbells, barbells, and movements.

THIRD WORKOUT DAY

On your third workout day, which should bring you into the next week, you will be ready to complete a full routine. Now you will do your first set at fifteen repetitions, just as you did before, and your second set with a heavier weight at ten repetitions. But now you will add the final set of six to eight repetitions at a still heavier weight. You will learn to judge which weights to use as you realize that the beginning weight must be heavy enough to present a challenge at fifteen repetitions, the next weight heavy enough to make you work hard for the ten repetitions, and the final and third weight for your set of six to eight repetitions must be heavy enough to make you say, "This is murder, but I can make it because I only have to get six reps." This graduated system makes sense because you will be sore, but not so sore that you will be tempted to quit.

SHOULD YOU WORK ALONE OR WITH A PARTNER?

The choice is yours. While a training partner can encourage some people, he or she can slow others down. If you work hard and fast and are self-disciplined, we suggest that you work without a partner. On the other hand, if you need a little push, why not find someone to work with. If you don't fall into the trap of talking during your workout, and if you make sure you do your set immediately after your partner finishes his or hers, a partner will not slow you down.

STRETCHING

The pyramid system provides a natural stretch for each muscle. As you will recall, you will be doing your first set of each exercise with a weight light enough to allow you to achieve fifteen repetitions.This light first set gives your working muscle a chance to warm up before you advance to the heavier second and third sets. If you wish to do some extra stretching, consult the bibliography for an excellent book that provides simple stretches for each bodypart (*Reach for It*, by Ardy Friedberg).

LOCATING YOUR MUSCLES

Before you actually get down to business, with or without a partner, you have to know where your muscles are located. Why? When you are working out, it is crucial that you keep your mind on the bodypart (the specific muscle) you are trying to develop. Here is a list of the muscles you should become acquainted with. After you have read the definition, look at the anatomy pictures (pp. 26–27) and then locate the muscle on your own body. Then, whenever you work out, think about the particular muscle you are exercising. Keep your mind on that muscle for every single repetition of that exercise. For example, if you are doing the bench press, realize that you are working your pectoral (chest) muscles and make these and not your arm muscles do the work. This is essential if the targeted muscle is going to receive the greatest possible benefit from doing a particular exercise.

BICEPS. Your biceps is located in the front of your upper arm, between your elbow and shoulder joint. It is your biceps that flexes your elbow joint.

TRICEPS. The three-headed triceps muscle travels along your upper arm. It is used to extend your forearm, and it is the muscle that commonly begins to sag after the age of thirty.

CHEST. Your chest muscles are located under your breasts. They are also called "pectorals." Your chest muscles assist you in moving your upper arms and, when developed, help to keep your breasts from sagging and to provide the attractive look of "cleavage."

SHOULDERS (deltoids). These three-headed muscles, located in your shoulders, help to raise your arm. The three aspects of this muscle are: front, side, and rear.

BACK. Your back consists of two main muscle groups. Your trapezius muscles and your latissimus dorsi, or "lats." Your trapezius muscles run on either side of your spine from the back of your neck to the middle of your back. They are used to support your head and to help raise your head and shoulders. You can see your traps from a front view by looking at the area between your neck and shoulders. Your latissimus dorsi muscles rise along your spinal column from the middle of your back to your tailbone. The lats give your back its width. When you begin to develop your lats, you will appear to have a smaller waist, because an athletic "V" look is produced. Your lats are used to help pull your shoulders back and your arms toward your body.

ABDOMINALS. Your abdominal, or "stomach," muscles consist of two main areas: upper and lower. They originate from the rib area near your breastbone and are used to help pull your torso toward your lower body. You will find that you use your abdominal muscles for nearly every exercise because it is from the abdominal area that your strength originates. Your upper abdominals are located between your waist and lower chest area, and your lower abdominals are located between your waist and pubic-bone area.

BUTTOCKS. Your buttocks, or "gluteus maximus," are the largest muscles in your body (as you may have noticed—especially if they have begun to sag and if

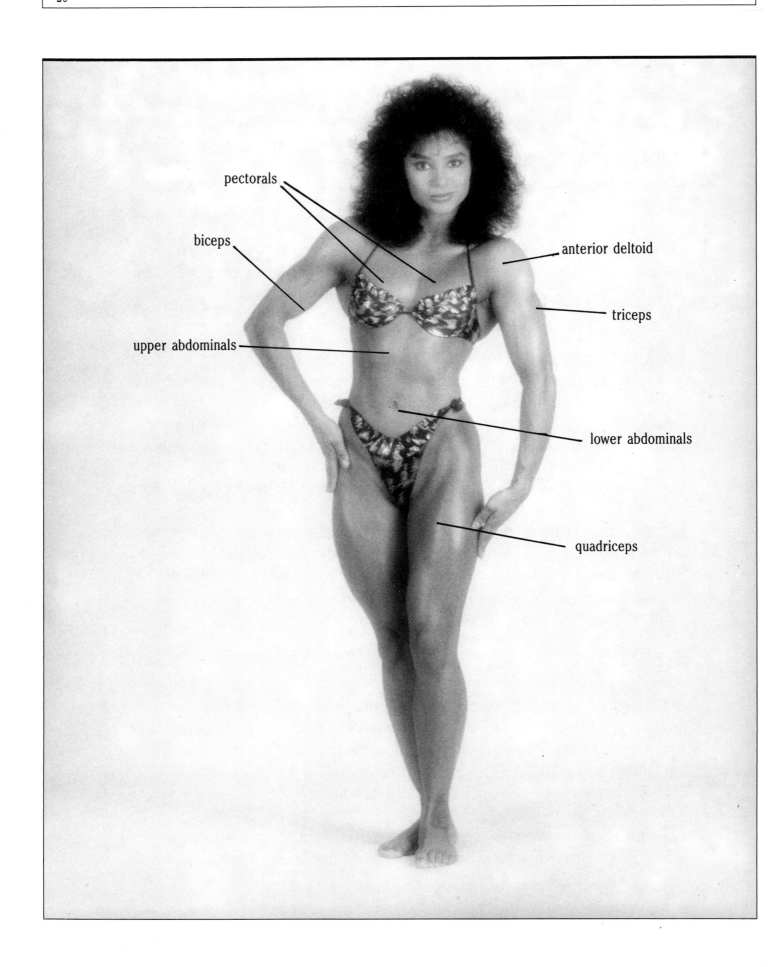

pectorals

biceps

anterior deltoid

triceps

upper abdominals

lower abdominals

quadriceps

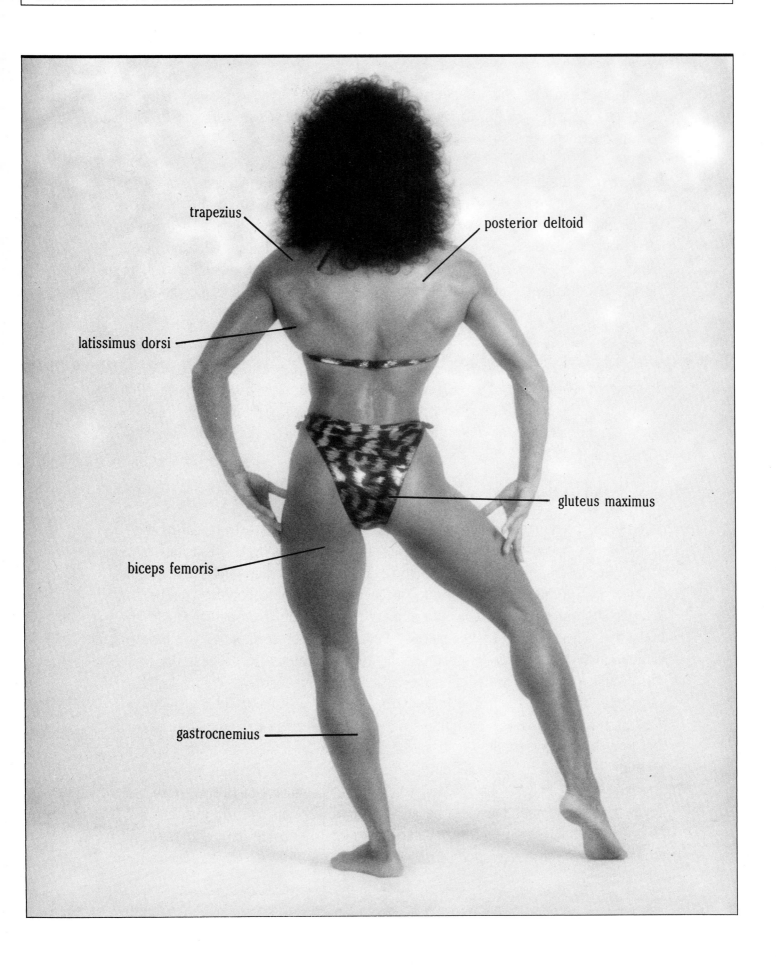

they have acquired a good amount of fat over them). These muscles originate in your back hipbone and run to your tailbone. They are used to help you extend and rotate your thigh.

LEGS. Your leg has three main muscle areas; your front thigh, or "quadriceps," your back thigh, or "biceps femoris" or "hamstrings," and your calf, or "gastrocnemius." Your quadriceps (front thigh) muscle is a large, four-part extensor muscle. Your biceps femoris (back thigh) is a two-headed muscle that flexes your knee, rotates your leg, and extends your hips. Your gastrocnemius (calf) muscle is a two-headed muscle that is used to flex your knee and foot downward.

HOW TO WORK WITH THE WEIGHTS

Because this program has been tailor-made for the busy woman, we have eliminated all of the frills. This means it is absolutely necessary for you to follow the program exactly. Only if you do this can we guarantee the result.

ISOLATION OF MUSCLES

In order to challenge the bodypart you are working, you have to do all of the exercises for that bodypart before advancing to the next bodypart. You must never skip from one bodypart to another. For example, notice that your chest routine consists of the flat bench press and the incline flye. Your shoulder routine consists of another two exercises, the military press to the front and the side lateral raise. (See pp. 71, 87 for exercise summary sheets.) Suppose you have just completed your bench press exercise and you just happen to be near the barbell with which you can do your military press, but you have not yet completed your other chest exercise, the incline flye. Sorry. You cannot, for convenience's sake or for any other reason, jump from a chest exercise to a shoulder exercise and then back again to chest and so on. This is not a hit-and-miss system. It is carefully designed to challenge and stress each bodypart. By going from one bodypart to another and back again, you remove the power of the exercises to develop and tone your muscles, because you give that muscle too long a rest. The muscle must continue to work hard in order to become hard and solid. So, *do all exercises for a given bodypart before advancing to those for another bodypart.*

THE PYRAMID SYSTEM

The basic principle of the pyramid system that you do three sets of each exercise, and that you "pyramid," or add weight to each set at the expense of a few reps, was discussed on p. 21. Now it's time to apply that principle to your own workout.

These are the numerical guidelines you should follow when using the pyramid technique:

Set 1. 12–15 reps (lightest weight)
Set 2. 8–10 reps (next heaviest weight)
Set 3. 6–8 reps (heaviest weight)

Select a weight for your first set that provides a challenge, but not a great struggle, when completing twelve to fifteen repetitions. Be sure that the weight you select is light enough to allow you to perform the exercise in perfectly strict form.

For your second set, select a slightly higher weight. For example, if you did your first set of the bench press with twenty-five pounds at fifteen repetitions, add ten pounds (five on each end of the bar) and do your second set of ten repetitions with thirty-five pounds. For your final, and heaviest, set, add another ten pounds and do your six to eight repetitions with forty-five pounds.

LEARNING ABOUT HOW MUCH WEIGHT TO ADD

You'll have to "fool around" with the weights a little in order to learn what your body can do. Don't get involved in proving something to yourself about how heavy you can go. The idea is to get used to the system and to perform the exercises in perfect form. Later on you can challenge yourself with heavier weights—as your body gets used to the system.

For example, using the bench press model, you may not be able to add a full ten pounds for your last set. If not, add a two-and-a-half-pound plate to each end of the barbell, making your last set forty pounds.

The main point is, *add weight to each set.*

WHAT IF THE NEXT AVAILABLE WEIGHT IS TOO HEAVY?

Suppose your home or gym equipment lacks various dumbbells, plates, or barbells? For example, say you have done your first bench press of fifteen repetitions at twenty-five pounds. You find five-pound plates and do your next set of ten repetitions at thirty-five pounds. But you can't manage to do forty-five pounds for your last set, and there are no two-and-a-half pound plates available to add to each end of the barbell. Simple. For the time being, just do your last set at the same weight, until you become strong enough to use the available weights and do your last set at forty-five pounds.

There's yet another way to go. You can try to use the too-heavy weight and get a minimum of four repetitions. This is okay when you are breaking into a new weight category.

The bottom line is, if the ideal weights are not available, work the equipment on hand with the goal of pyramiding each set in the very near future. You'll surprise yourself with the strength you build in a very short time.

PROGRESSION

After you have been working out for a few weeks, you may find that it is too easy to lift the weights you are using. When this happens, it is time to raise your weights—for each set. Start with a heavier weight and add weight to each set. For example, in the bench press example, if you used to do:

Set 1. 12–15 reps, 25 pounds
Set 2. 8–10 reps, 35 pounds
Set 3. 6–8 reps, 45 pounds

Now do:

Set 1. 12–15 reps, 35 pounds
Set 2. 8–10 reps, 45 pounds
Set 3. 6–8 reps, 55 pounds

Again, if you can't make the added weight for the last set, follow the suggestions previously discussed.

FOLLOWING THE ROUTINE

In the beginning, it is a good idea to follow the routine exactly as given. Later on (after about three months), you can change things around in the following ways (and only in the following ways).

CHANGING THE ORDER OF EXERCISES WITHIN A BODYPART

There is nothing sacred about the order within a bodypart group. For example, in the chest routine, although the flat bench press is listed before the incline flye, there is no reason you can't do the incline flye *before* the bench press if you wish. In the shoulder routine, although the military press to the front is listed first, you can do the side lateral raise first, and so on.

CHANGING THE ORDER OF THE BODYPARTS

There is also nothing sacred about the order of the bodyparts in your workout. For example, we have instructed you to do your chest first, your shoulders, then your back, then your biceps, triceps, legs, buttocks, and abdominals. You can change that around in any way you please. You may want to get your legs out of the way first, since you may dread working them. You may decide to do your abdominals first because they are used in almost every exercise. You may be the kind of person who likes to do the easy things first—to ease gradually into the workout. If so, you may find your back a good place to start. It is generally better to work the most difficult or troublesome bodyparts first.

We advise that you keep the order given here for the first three months—until you get used to the exercises and until you get to know your own body. After that, you can do anything you please, as long as you keep the exercises within the bodypart and as long as you do your three sets for each exercise and re-member to pyramid the weights.

USING THIS BOOK

In the beginning, you will have to take this book to the gym and follow the pictures and instructions for every exercise. After about a month, you will no longer need to carry the book around. You'll remember your routine. However, for your convenience, we have provided a list of all the exercises at the end of the workout chapter. This exercise summary sheet can be copied and taken to the gym so that you can check off your exercises as you go along.

SUMMARY OF HOW TO USE THE WEIGHTS

- Do each bodypart in isolation of other bodyparts. Never mix bodyparts.
- Do three sets for each bodypart. Add weight to each set while decreasing the number of repetitions. The formula is:

    Set 1. 12–15 reps
    Set 2. 8–10 reps
    Set 3. 6–8 reps

- Be patient with yourself as you learn how much weight to use and how much weight to add.
- When your beginning weight becomes too easy, add weight to each set.
- After three months, you can change the order within a bodypart as well as the order of the bodyparts you work.
- After three months you may try some of the "For a change" alternate exercises, included with each exercise.
- After one month, all you will need is the workout summary sheet on pages 71 or 87.

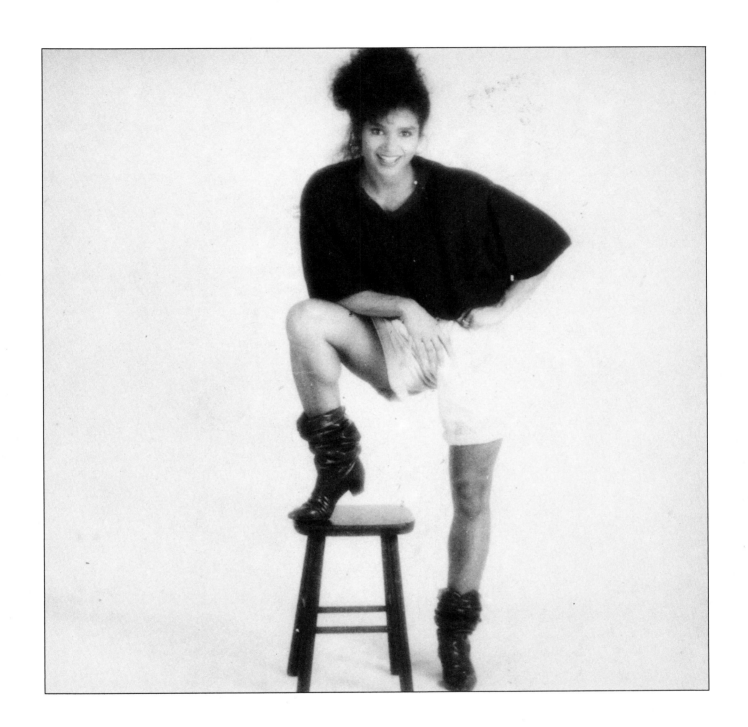

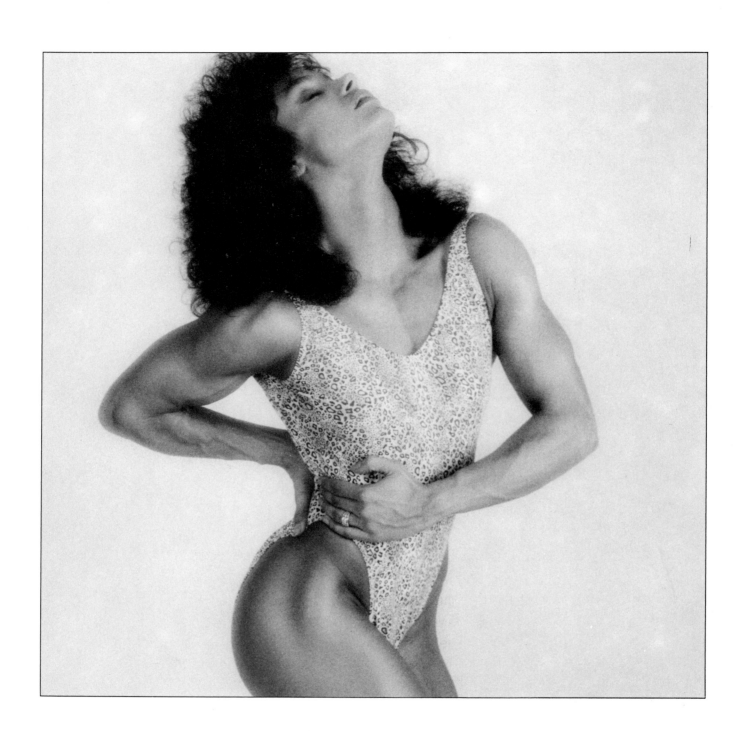

HARD BODIES EXPRESS GYM WORKOUT

If you have chosen to work out in the gym, you probably did so because of the following advantages.

- None of the distractions of the home (like the telephone) are present to lure you away from the work at hand.
- You can gain from the encouragement of other people who are working toward the same goal as you.
- There will be a wide variety of equipment available to you.
- You don't have to see the gym equipment at home. When you leave the gym, you leave it all behind until the next workout.
- You can take advantage of "spotters" and "training partners."
- You can meet new friends, both male and female.
- You are likely to go because you've paid your yearly membership fee and do not want to see it go to waste.

The following pages describe your workout step-by-step. Follow the instructions and pictures exactly as you see them. Do not try any of the variations until you have been working out for at least three months.

Once you know how to do your exercises correctly without looking at the book, you might want to take advantage of the workout summary sheet provided at the end of this chapter. As I mentioned before, it lists the entire workout. You make a Xerox copy of it to bring to the gym with you.

WHICH GYM SHOULD I JOIN?

The ideal gym for this workout is one that has a variety of free weights. As you will notice, this workout requires more use of free weights than machines.

Free weights force you to do *all* of the work. Machines take some of the stress away from you. What is more, it is much easier to cheat with a machine, since you know that the machine will "catch" the weight if you become sloppy in your techniques. The only time we ask you to use a machine is when there is no equivalent free weight exercise. For example, it is impossible to create perfect lats without the use of the lat machine. While there are good substitutions, the lat machine is really the best way to develop lats.

However, it is a good idea to experiment with the machine substitutes once in a while for the sake of variety. For example, if you usually do your bench press on the free weight bench press station, once in a while you can use the Universal Gym or other machine bench press. Today there are hundreds of brand-name machinery, so don't be concerned with whether the machine says Paragon, Nautilus, Cybex, Universal, or any other name.

Most gyms that stress free weights are gyms that stress bodybuilding as opposed to general fitness. In such gyms you are likely to find a minimum of "fringes" such as swimming pools, steam rooms, saunas, and juice bars. In fact, you will probably see a rather rudimentary setup. A nonrugged floor is not unusual. The weights, the machines, and a simple shower are all that serious bodybuilders are concerned with.

In such a gym, you will notice that people do not hold conversations while they work out. Their minds are on what they are doing. Such an atmosphere encourages strict concentration and results in increased progress. For this reason, joining such a gym is not a bad idea, even though you do have to give up some of the frills. On the up side, these gyms usually have much lower yearly membership fees.

You might be someone, however, who enjoys the frills. You want to feel "pampered." You love the idea of a hot sauna or whirlpool session after your workout and you can't wait to hit the juice bar. Great. There's no reason why you can't join such a varied facility. Just make sure they have plenty of free weights, and that they let you follow your own (this) program. If they insist on everyone who joins being instructed by their personnel and having to follow their programs, forget it. You'll be in the same dilemma as thousands of other women who are spending hours in gyms and seeing little results.

The crucial point is, join a gym where you can freely follow this program with a minimum of interference.

CHEST ROUTINE

FLAT BENCH PRESS—CHEST EXERCISE #1

DEVELOPS, SHAPES, TONES:
- Pectoral (chest) muscles that uphold the breasts.

GET READY
- Lie on a flat exercise bench. Position your shoulders just under the barbell.

ACTION:
- Grip the bar about 6 inches wider than shoulder width and lift it out of its holding device. Hold it straight up with your arms fully extended above you.
- Lower the bar until it grazes your chest. Stretch your chest.
- Raise the bar to start position and flex your chest.
- Repeat this movement without resting until you have completed your set.

CAREFUL:
- Maintain a steady pace—not too fast, not too slow.
- Control the barbell. Don't become lazy and let it drop onto your chest. Keep your head flat on the bench and centered.
- Be sure you have a balanced grip before you start the exercise. A lopsided barbell produces haphazard results.
- Concentrate on your chest muscles. Work with your chest, not your arms.

FOR A CHANGE:
- Do this exercise on a decline bench. It will especially develop your lower chest area. (You may place an 8- to 16-inch block of wood under a bench if no decline bench is available.)
- Do this exercise on an incline bench. It will especially develop your upper breast area.
- Do this exercise on a decline bench with dumbbells.

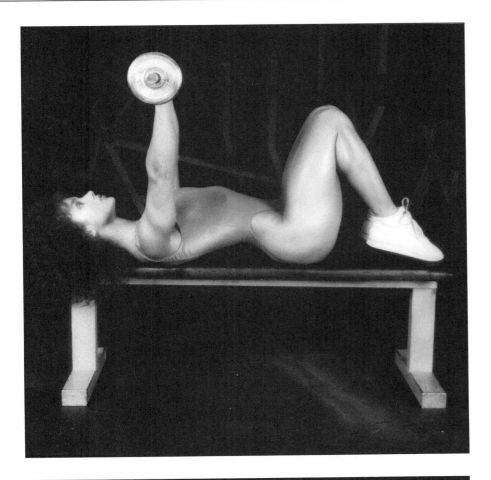

FLAT BENCH PRESS (START)

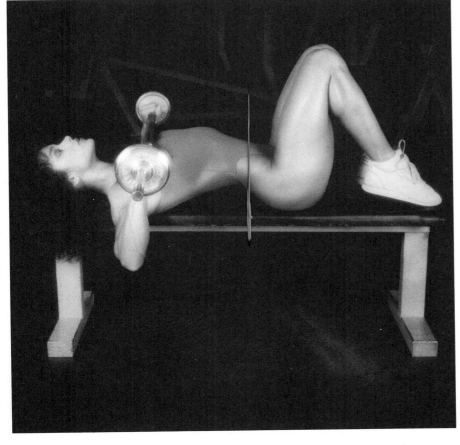

FLAT BENCH PRESS (FINISH)

INCLINE FLYE—CHEST EXERCISE #2

DEVELOPS, SHAPES, TONES:	• Upper pectoral (breast) muscles that produce the look of cleavage.
GET READY:	• Lie on an incline bench with one dumbbell in each hand. • Extend your arms over your head so that the dumbbells are held in line with your shoulder joints. • Position your palms to face each other.
ACTION:	• Move your arms outward and downward in a semicircle. You will have to bend your arms slightly at the elbow. • Continue to move on the semicircle until you feel a full stretch in your pectoral (chest) area. • Return to starting position and repeat the movement until you have completed your set.
CAREFUL:	• Don't let your back rise off the flat of the bench. • Flex (squeeze) your pectoral muscles on the upward movement and stretch them on the downward movement. • Control the weights at all times. Never let the dumbbells drop quickly to the down position. Never jerk them up to the start position. • Keep your mind on the bodypart you are working. Think chest, not arms.
FOR A CHANGE:	• Do this exercise on a flat exercise bench. It will develop the entire breast (pectoral) area.

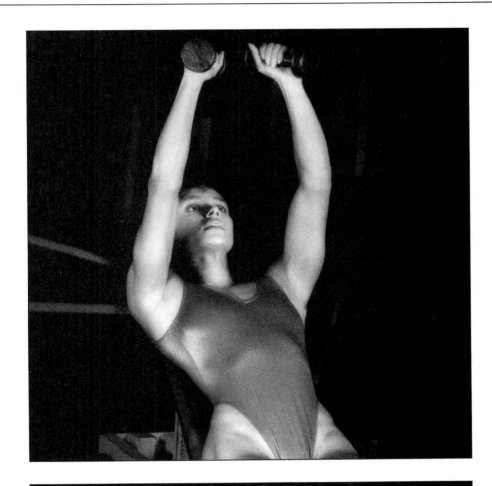

INCLINE FLYE (START)

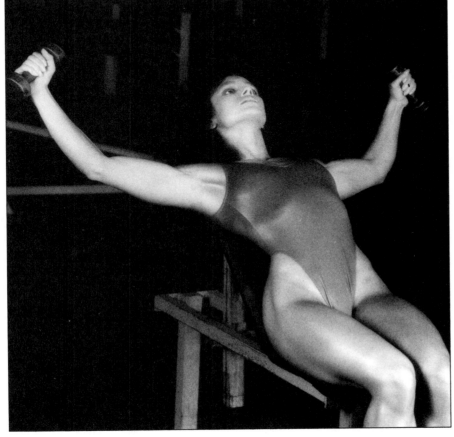

INCLINE FLYE (FINISH)

SHOULDER ROUTINE

MILITARY PRESS TO THE REAR—SHOULDER EXERCISE #1

DEVELOPS, SHAPES, TONES:
- Front deltoid (shoulder) muscles.
- Trapezius muscles (connecting your neck and shoulders).

GET READY:
- Stand with your feet a natural width apart.
- Hold a barbell, palms away from you, with your hands about 6 inches wider than shoulder width.
- Hold the barbell so that it rests on your shoulders and trapezius muscles.

ACTION:
- Raise the barbell straight up until your arms are fully extended.
- Return to start position.
- Repeat the movement until you have completed your set.

CAREFUL:
- Flex (squeeze together) your shoulder muscles on the up movement and stretch them on the down movement.
- Keep your mind on your front shoulder muscles. Make those muscles do the work.
- Never jerk the barbell up, and maintain control while returning to start position.

FOR A CHANGE:
- Do the exercise while seated. It is more difficult, but your shoulders work harder.
- Do the exercise holding the barbell on your upper chest muscles. This method is slightly more difficult than the rear military press. You may do it standing or seated.

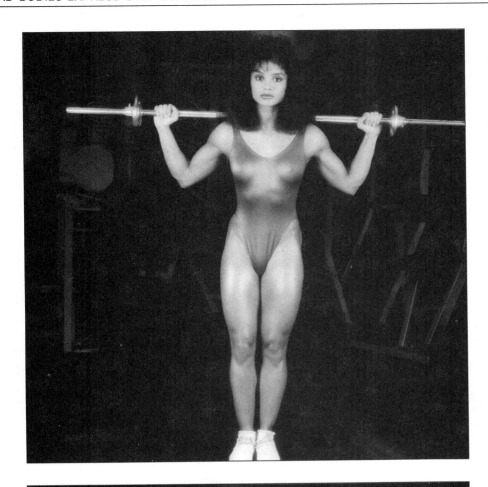

MILITARY PRESS TO THE REAR
(START)

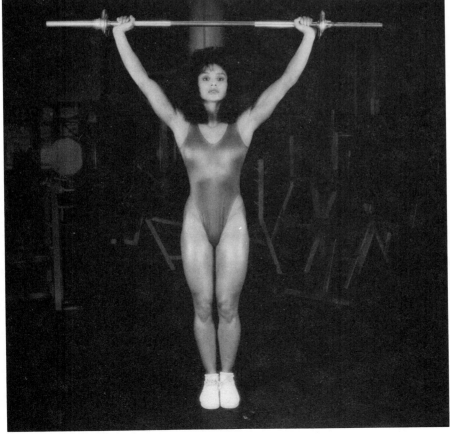

MILITARY PRESS TO THE REAR
(FINISH)

SIDE LATERAL RAISE—SHOULDER EXERCISE #2

DEVELOPS, SHAPES, TONES:	• Side deltoid (shoulder) muscles. • The trapezius muscles (see anatomy chart p. 27).
GET READY:	• Stand with your feet a natural width apart. • Hold one dumbbell in each hand with your palms facing each other. • Hold the dumbbells in front of you at the center of your body. Let them touch. • Lean forward very slightly. Maintain a comfortable stance.
ACTION:	• Raise the dumbbells away from your body until they are at ear height. You will have to bend your elbows slightly. • Return to start position and repeat the movement until you have completed your set.
CAREFUL:	• Control the dumbbells at all times. • Flex your shoulders on the up movement and stretch them on the down movement. • Don't swing your arms. Let your shoulders do the work. • Watch your shoulder (deltoid) muscles working in the mirror.
FOR A CHANGE:	• Lie on an incline bench and perform the movement with one arm at a time. Do all the reps for one set with one arm and then switch to the other arm. This forces you to work each shoulder equally hard. • Do the exercise seated. It is more difficult, but your shoulders work harder.

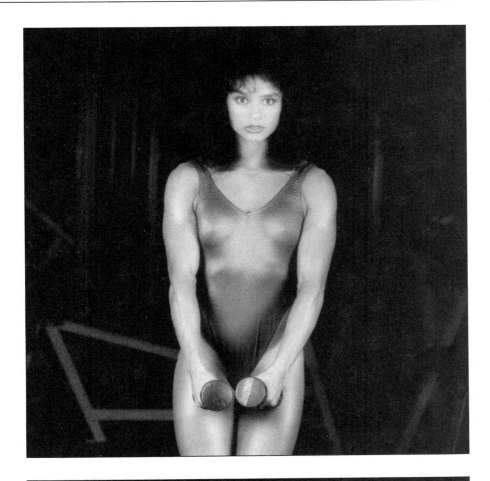

SIDE LATERAL RAISE
(START)

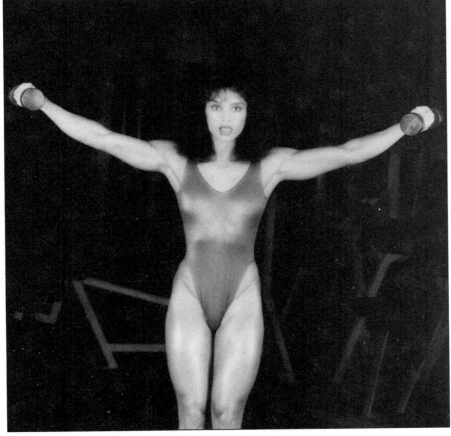

SIDE LATERAL RAISE
(FINISH)

BACK ROUTINE

LAT MACHINE PULLDOWN TO THE REAR—BACK EXERCISE #1

DEVELOPS, SHAPES, TONES:

- Lats, or back, muscles (latissimus dorsi). Gives your back the athletic "V" look and makes your waist appear smaller.

GET READY:

- Sit in the machine seat of any lat pulldown machine.

- Adjust the seat to a comfortable position.

- Grip the bar lat pulldown with your hands 2 inches away from the down-curve end of the bar. Keep your palms facing forward.

- Extend your arms fully upward and let the weight of the bar stretch out your back. Lean forward.

ACTION:

- Pull the bar down until it touches your trapezius and shoulder area. Make sure you pull with your latissimus dorsi muscles and not with your arms.

- Return to start position and repeat the movement until you have completed your set.

CAREFUL:

- Never let the bar pull you up. Control the weights. Let the weights stretch you on each up movement.

- Never jerk the bar down. Move it in full control. Flex (squeeze together) your latissimus dorsi muscles on the down movement.

FOR A CHANGE:

- Do this exercise to the front. Lower the bar to your upper chest.

- Vary your grip. Use a narrow grip (about 6 inches wider than shoulder width.

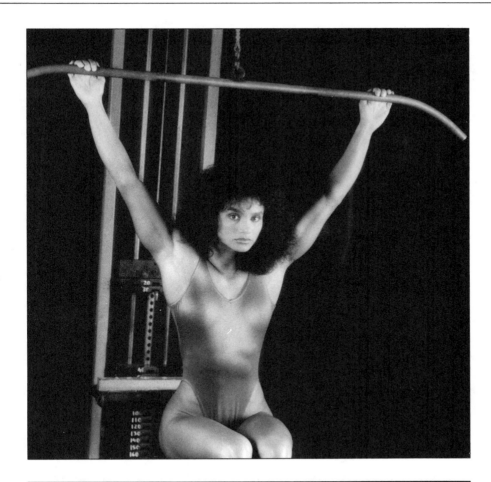

LAT MACHINE PULLDOWN
TO THE REAR (START)

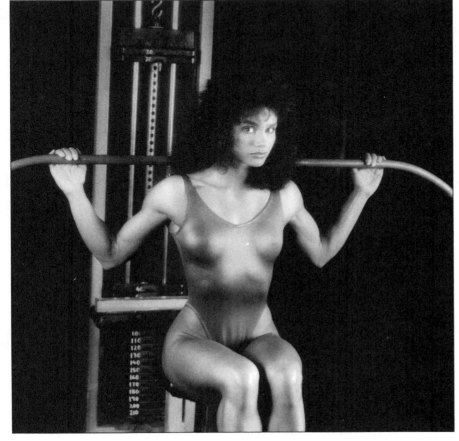

LAT MACHINE PULLDOWN
TO THE REAR (FINISH)

PULLEY ROW—BACK EXERCISE #2

DEVELOPS, SHAPES, TONES:	• Upper back area.
	• Latissimus dorsi (lats) muscles.
GET READY:	• Sit at the pulley machine.
	• Place your feet against the footrest and bend your knees slightly.
	• Grip the pulley and lean forward. Let your back stretch out.
ACTION:	• Pull the handles to your *waist* while you rise to a perpendicular position. Flex your back. Throw your chest out.
	• Return to start position. Let the weights stretch out your back.
	• Repeat the movement until you have completed your set.
CAREFUL:	• Don't do the work with your arms. Use your lat muscles.
	• Never jerk the weights to your waist. Control them.
	• Never let the weights pull you forward. Slowly return to start each time.
FOR A CHANGE:	• Pull the weights to your *lower chest* area. This will help develop your upper back muscles rather than your latissimus dorsi muscles.

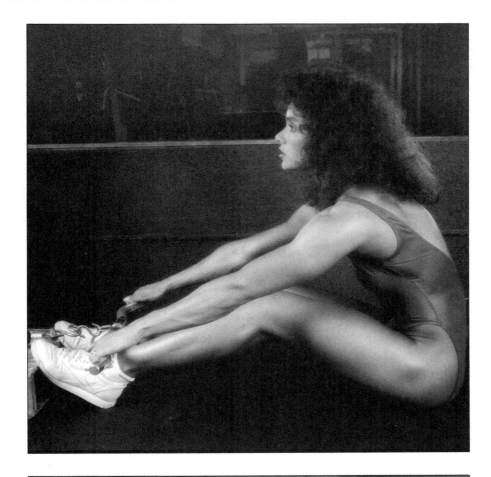

PULLEY ROW (START)

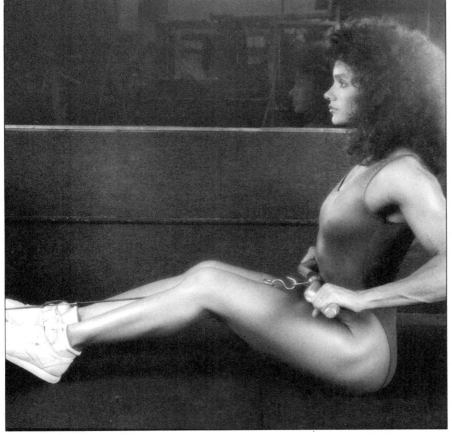

PULLEY ROW (FINISH)

BICEPS ROUTINE

SEATED ALTERNATING BICEPS CURL—BICEPS EXERCISE #1

DEVELOPS, SHAPES, TONES:	• Entire biceps area.
GET READY:	• Sit at the edge of a flat exercise bench. Face the mirror.
	• Hold a dumbbell in each hand with your palms facing the mirror.
	• Sit up straight and keep your arms straight down at your sides.
ACTION:	• Raise your right arm to shoulder height until the dumbbell can go no higher. While you are lowering the dumbbell to start position, begin to raise the left arm to shoulder height and do so until that dumbbell can go no higher.
	• Continue this alternate up-down movement until you have completed your set.
CAREFUL:	• Keep your inner arms pinned to your upper body throughout the movement.
	• Never jerk the dumbbells up or let them drop. Control the weights.
	• Remember to flex (squeeze) your biceps on the up movement and to stretch them out on the down movement.
	• Be careful not to let your back or shoulders do the work. Your back should remain still. Do not sway at all. Throw your mind into your biceps.
FOR A CHANGE:	• Do this exercise standing. It is easier, but you can use heavier weights.
	• Do this exercise by curling both arms at the same time. You can do both arms at the same time standing or sitting.
	• Do the exercise standing but use a barbell instead of dumbbells.

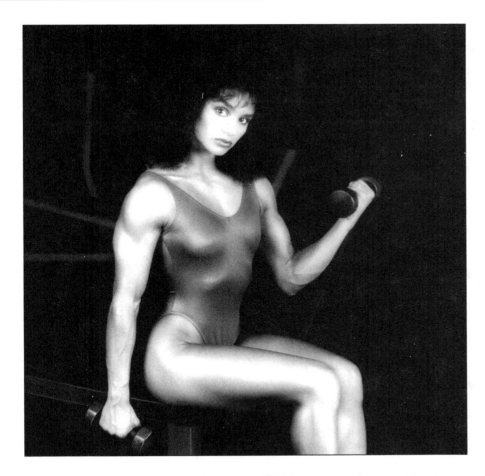

ALTERNATING BICEPS CURL
(START)

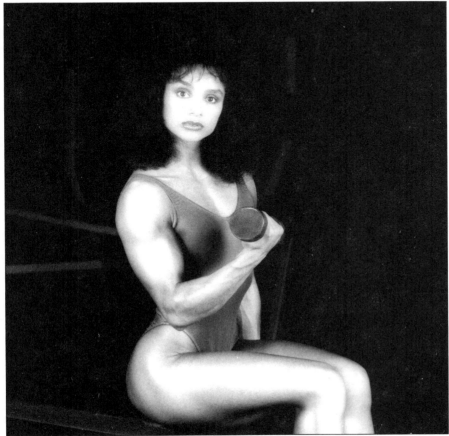

ALTERNATING BICEPS CURL
(FINISH)

CONCENTRATION CURL—BICEPS EXERCISE #2

DEVELOPS, SHAPES, TONES:

- The peak (head) of the biceps muscle.

GET READY:

- Sit on a flat exercise bench.
- Place your feet a comfortable width apart and grasp a dumbbell in your right hand.
- Lean forward at the waist. Place your right elbow on your right inner knee. Hold the dumbbell with your palm facing away from you.
- Keep your arm straight down.

ACTION:

- Keep your wrist locked and curl your arm upward. Keep your eye on your biceps muscle.
- Return to start. Do not sit up. Keep your position.
- Repeat the movement until you have completed your set.
- Do the exercise for the other arm.

CAREFUL:

- Don't try to use a heavy weight. Even powerlifters use relatively light weights for this exercise.
- Flex (squeeze) your biceps on the up movement and stretch them on the down movement.
- Don't sit up during the set. Keep your position.
- Never swing the dumbbell up or let it nearly drop down. Control the weight at all times.

FOR A CHANGE:

- Do the exercise standing up and leaning forward. You'll be forced to keep your position.

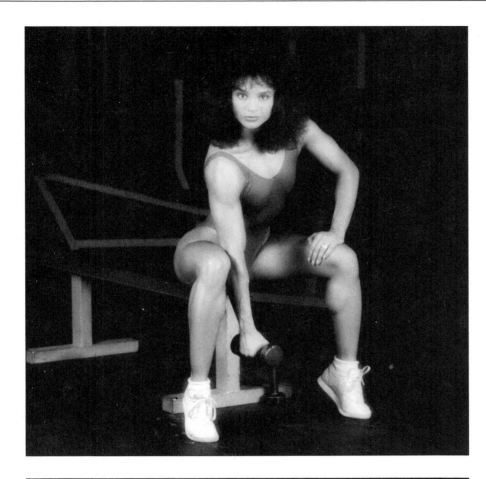

CONCENTRATION CURL
(START)

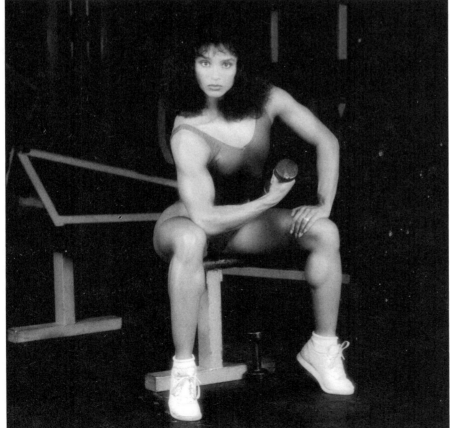

CONCENTRATION CURL
(FINISH)

TRICEPS ROUTINE

PULLEY PUSHDOWN—TRICEPS EXERCISE #1

DEVELOPS, SHAPES, TONES:	• Outer area of the triceps muscle. Entire triceps muscle.
GET READY:	• Place a pulley pushdown bar on any appropriate pulley device. • Place your hands, palms away from you, about 6 to 8 inches apart. • Bend your elbows and keep your upper arms close to your body.
ACTION:	• Push the bar down until you can go no farther. • Return to start position. • Repeat the movement until you have performed the correct number of repetitions for your set.
CAREFUL:	• Never let your elbows wander outward. Pin them to your sides. • Never let the weight pull you up. Control it at all times. • Never jerk the bar down. Concentrate. • Keep your mind on your triceps muscle throughout the exercise.
FOR A CHANGE:	• You may use a straight bar and keep your hands about 6 inches apart.

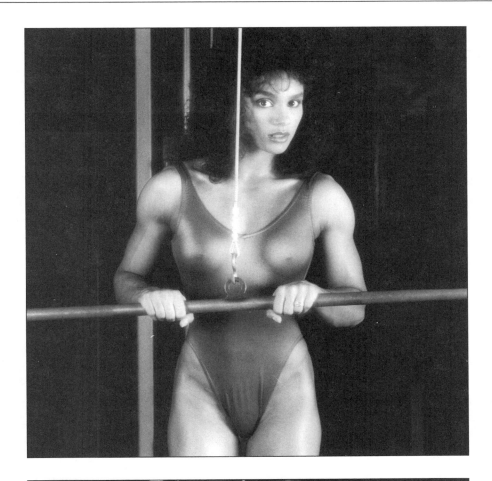

PULLEY PUSHDOWN (START)

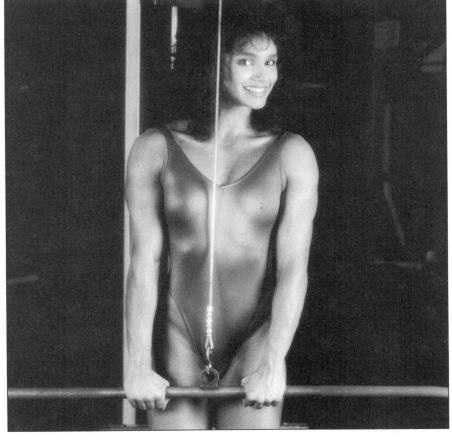

PULLEY PUSHDOWN (FINISH)

ONE-ARM TRICEPS EXTENSION—TRICEPS EXERCISE #2

DEVELOPS, SHAPES, TONES:

- The middle area of the triceps muscle.

GET READY:

- Hold a dumbbell in your right hand and face the mirror.

- Raise your right arm straight up. Keep your biceps pinned to your ear. Your palm is facing the mirror.

- Keep your left arm straight down or around your waist (out of the way).

ACTION:

- Lower the dumbbell behind you until it touches the back of your neck.

- Raise the dumbbell to start position and repeat the movement until you have completed your set.

- Repeat the set for your left arm. Alternate between arms for each of your three sets.

CAREFUL:

- Never let your biceps move away from your ear.

- Concentrate on working your triceps muscle. Flex on the up movement and stretch on the down movement.

- Never let the weight nearly drop down. Control it.

- Never jerk the weight up. Concentrate.

FOR A CHANGE:

- Do this exercise with one dumbbell (a heavier one). Hold the dumbbell with both hands and perform the same basic movement.

- Do this exercise with a barbell, using both hands.

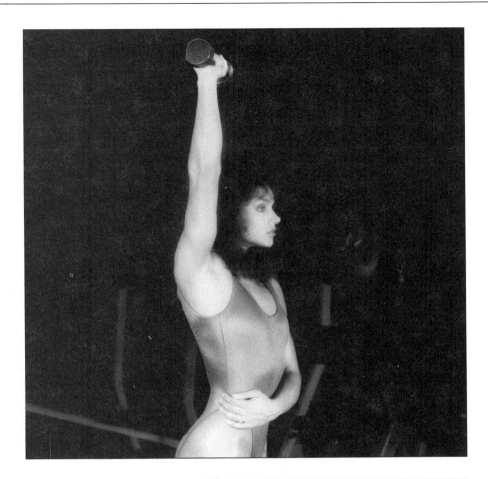

ONE-ARM TRICEPS EXTENSION (START)

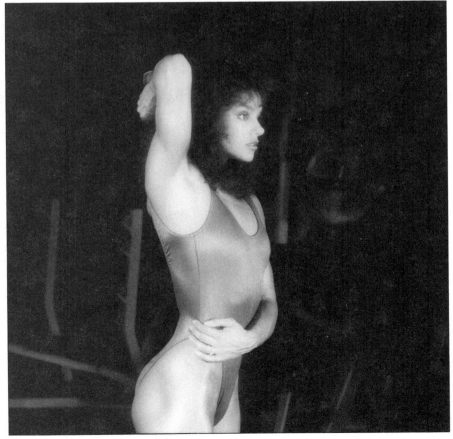

ONE-ARM TRICEPS EXTENSION (FINISH)

LEG EXTENSION—LEG EXERCISE #1

DEVELOPS, SHAPES, TONES:	• Front quadriceps (thigh) muscle.
GET READY:	• Sit in the seat of the leg extension machine, placing your insteps under the roller pads, or sit at the edge of an exercise bench wearing ankle weights. • Keep your back erect. • Grasp the handles or the bench on either side of you.
ACTION:	• Extend your legs until they are parallel to the floor. • Flex (squeeze) your front thigh (quadriceps) muscles and return to start position in full control of the weights. • Repeat the movement until you have completed your set.
CAREFUL:	• Never thrust your legs forward on the up movement. Control the weight at all times. • Don't allow your legs merely to drop back to start position. The downward movement is just as important as the upward movement. • Do not give in to the desire to rest between repetitions. Complete your set. • Watch your quadriceps muscles work as you flex them on the up movement. Envision your perfectly formed legs.
FOR A CHANGE:	• Do this exercise while lying down. Perform the movements in exactly the same manner as described above, only lie flat on your back. This position will help to develop your upper quadriceps muscle and will add attractive definition to that area. *Note:* Many gyms do not have a leg extension machine that allows the lying-down position. If this is the case, you will have to resort to performing the exercise with the ankle weights.

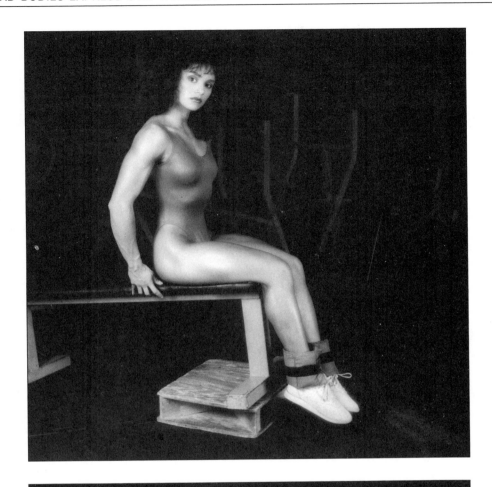

LEG EXTENSION (START)

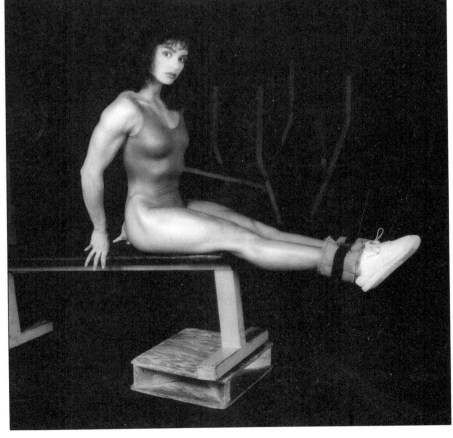

LEG EXTENSION (FINISH)

SQUAT—LEG EXERCISE #2

DEVELOPS, SHAPES, TONES:
- Quadriceps (front thigh) muscles.
- Gluteus maximus (buttocks) muscles.
- Hamstrings (back thigh muscles).

GET READY:
- Balance a barbell on your trapezius (upper rear shoulder) muscles.
- Stand with your feet a natural width apart, toes pointing slightly outward.
- Stand erect and look in the mirror in front of you.
- Keep your head and back straight throughout the exercise.

ACTION:
- Lower yourself into a squat. Keep your knees in line with your toes.
- Descend as low as you can and rise to start position. Repeat the movement until you have completed your set.

CAREFUL:
- Don't bounce up to start. Instead keep working hard. Control the weight.
- Do not lean forward. Keep your body as erect as possible.
- Flex your quadriceps on the up movement and stretch them on the down movement.
- You can place a 2-by-4 piece of wood under your heels to help give you balance.

FOR A CHANGE:
- Do this exercise to the front. Cross your arms in front of you and hold the barbell on your crossed arms.
- If you have never exercised your legs before, you may find that even the lightest weight on the leg extension machine is too heavy for you to lift. Since this is often the case, we have illustrated the exercise with ankle weights. Do the exercise with the ankle weights until your quadriceps muscles are strong enough to use the machine weights. (This should take no longer than six weeks.)

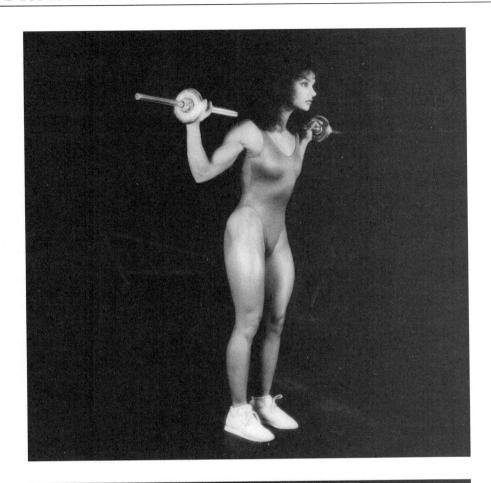

SQUAT (START)

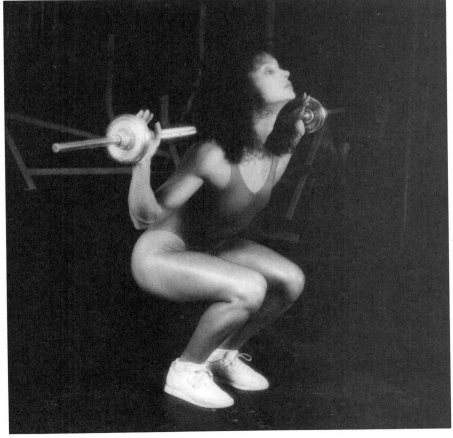

SQUAT (FINISH)

BUTTOCKS-HIP ROUTINE

FEATHER KICK-UP—BUTTOCKS-HIP EXERCISE #1

DEVELOPS, SHAPES, TONES:

- Lifts lower buttocks.
- Narrows buttocks-hip area.
- Tightens entire buttocks area.

GET READY:

- Get into an "all-fours" position on a flat exercise bench.
- Form your right leg into the shape of an "L." Your thigh should be parallel to the floor and to your body.

ACTION:

- Extend your leg upward using only the buttocks-to-thigh area.
- Straighten your leg and lift it as high as possible.
- Squeeze your buttocks on the up movement.
- Return to start and repeat the movement until you have completed your set.
- Repeat the set for the other leg. Continue to alternate legs until you have completed your three sets.

CAREFUL:

- This exercise is awkward in the beginning. Keep at it. In time it will become natural. It's very effective and worth the effort.
- Don't forget to flex your buttocks on the up movement.
- Never let your knee move from its high "L" position. Be aware of your leg's tendency to want to move downward toward the bench.
- Don't cut the movement short. Raise your leg as high as possible.

FOR A CHANGE:

- Do this exercise exactly as described. See "Express Training" for additional buttocks exercises.

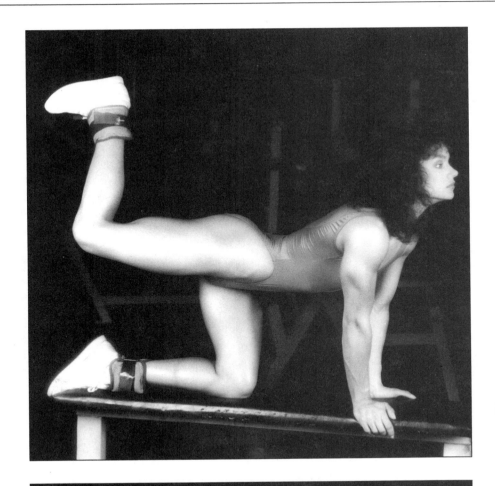

FEATHER KICK-UP (START)

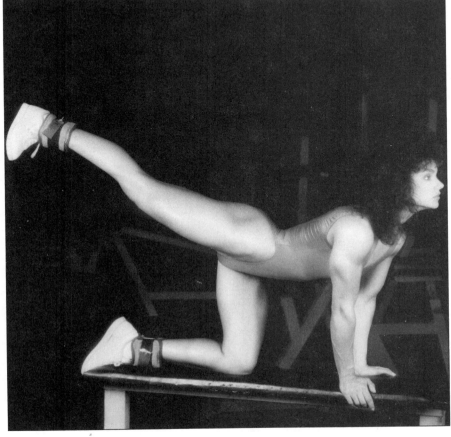

FEATHER KICK-UP (FINISH)

BENCH SCISSORS—BUTTOCKS-HIP EXERCISE #2

DEVELOPS, SHAPES, TONES:	• Entire buttocks area.

GET READY:

• Place ankle weights on your ankles and sit at the edge of a flat exercise bench.

• Grasp the sides of the bench or place your hands under your buttocks. Extend your legs out in front of you. Keep your buttocks close to the end of the bench.

• Lock your knees. Touch your ankles to each other. Flex (squeeze, tighten) your buttocks to keep them that way throughout the exercise.
Note: Many people think this is a leg exercise. It is not. It is crucial that you keep your buttocks flexed throughout the movement in order to achieve the buttocks-tightening and -lifting effect.

ACTION:

• Flex your buttocks and extend your legs outward as far as possible.

• Do not pause. Return to start and repeat the movement until you have completed your set.

CAREFUL:

• Flex. Flex. Flex.

• Do not cut the movement short. Go as wide as possible.

• Do not cross your legs over. Return to ankle-touching position each time.

• Keep your hands on the bench, under your buttocks, so you can feel the continual "flex."

FOR A CHANGE:

• You may do this exercise on an appropriate pulley machine.

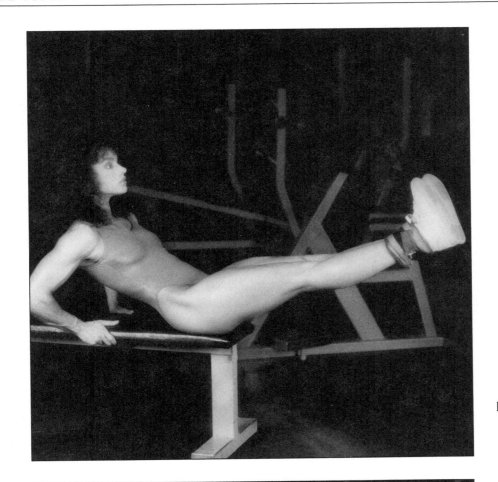

BENCH SCISSORS (START)

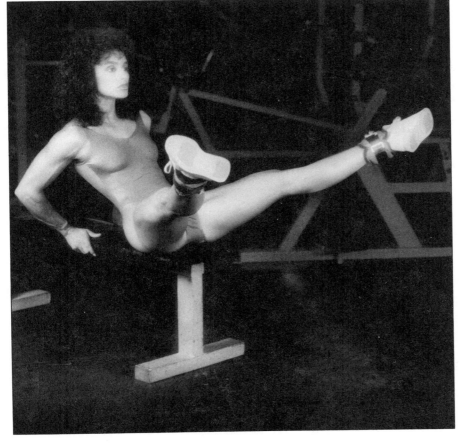

BENCH SCISSORS (FINISH)

ABDOMINAL ROUTINE

SIT-UP—ABDOMINAL EXERCISE #1

DEVELOPS, SHAPES, TONES:
- Upper abdominal area.

GET READY:
- Lie flat on your back. You may use the floor, a sit-up board, a mat, etc. Place your feet under a holding device if one is available.
- Bend your knees. Get your arms out of the way. Place them crossed over your chest or locked behind your neck.

ACTION:
- Slowly rise until you are perpendicular to the floor.
- Do not rest. Return to start and repeat the movement until you have completed your set.

CAREFUL:
- Never bounce off the start position. Squeeze your abdominal muscles and, in control, rise to perpendicular position.
- Never drop to start position. Keep your abdominal muscles flexed and return to start.
- Be aware that your abdominal muscles must be flexed throughout the entire exercise.

FOR A CHANGE:
- Do the exercise from side to side. Lock your hands behind your neck and bring each elbow to the opposite knee. (Left elbow to right knee, right elbow to left knee.)
- Do this exercise on an incline sit-up board.
- Do this exercise on a hyperextension bench, holding a 25-pound plate.

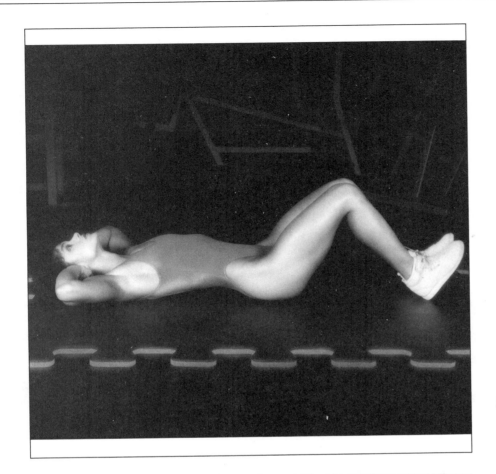

SIT-UP (START)

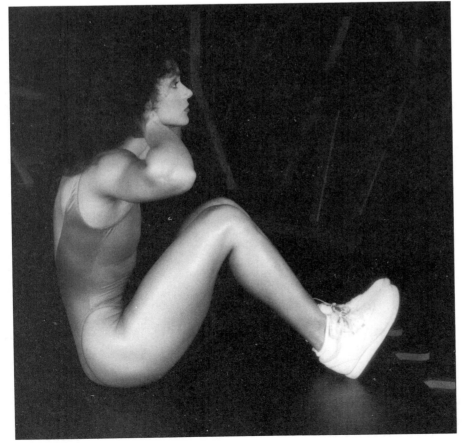

SIT-UP (FINISH)

LEG RAISE—ABDOMINAL EXERCISE #2

DEVELOPS, SHAPES, TONES:	• Lower abdominal area.
GET READY:	• Lie on a flat surface—the floor, a padded exercise board, a mat, a flat exercise bench, etc. • Place your hands next to or under your buttocks. • Extend your legs out in front of you. Flex your lower abdominals.
ACTION:	• Raise your legs until they are approximately perpendicular to the floor. • Keep your abdominals flexed. Return to start and repeat the movement until you have completed your set. Do not rest until you have completed the set.
CAREFUL:	• Keep your mind on your lower abdominals. Flex them hard throughout the exercise. • Don't swing your legs up or let them drop down. Control your movements.
FOR A CHANGE:	• Do this exercise with a light weight held between your feet.

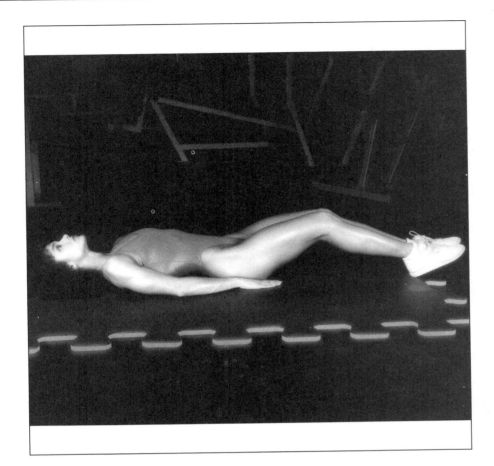

LEG RAISE
(START)

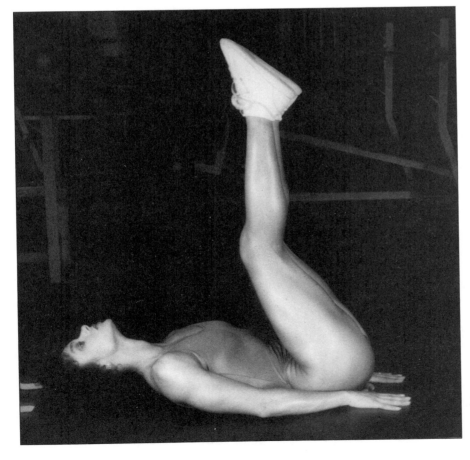

LEG RAISE
(FINISH)

REMINDERS

- Flex (squeeze, tighten).
- Stretch (expand, extend).
- Keep your mind on the bodypart you are working.
- Do not cut the movement short.
- Never jerk the weight up.
- Do not let the weight drop quickly to start position.
- Do not rest during a set.
- Do not pyramid the weights on buttocks and abdominals.
- Work your way up to 3 sets of 25 or 50 repetitions on all buttocks and abdominal exercises.
- When the initial weight becomes too easy, raise your weights.
- Continually picture your body evolving into the perfect body you have in mind.
- You may try some of the "for a change" alternates after training for three months.

WORKOUT SUMMARY

Chest
1. Flat Bench Press
2. Incline Flye

Shoulder
1. Military Press to the Rear
2. Side Lateral Raise

Back
1. Lat Machine Pulldown to the Rear
2. Pulley Row

Biceps
1. Seated Alternate Biceps Curl
2. Concentration Curl

Triceps
1. Pulley Pushdown
2. One-arm Triceps Extension

Leg routine
1. Leg Extension
2. Squat

Buttocks-hip
1. Feather Kick-up
2. Bench scissors

Abdominals
1. Sit-up
2. Leg Raise

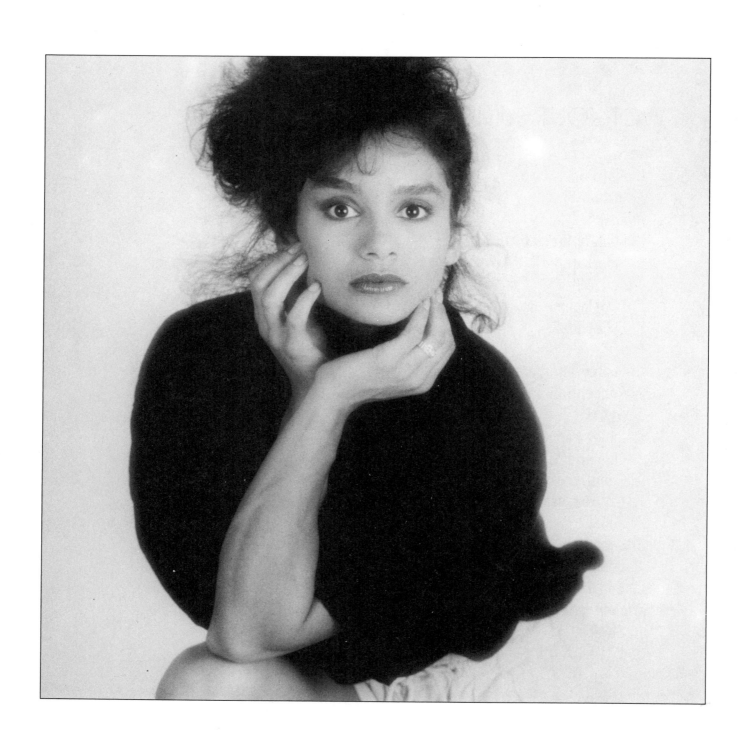

HARD BODIES EXPRESS HOME WORKOUT

There are several distinct advantages to working out at home. If you have chosen the home workout, perhaps you have done so for the following reasons.

- You can work out without the distraction of people around you.
- You can choose your own workout times—anytime, day or night.
- You save time in travel.
- You save money in the long run. Your investment for gym equipment is less than the price of a yearly gym membership.
- You have complete privacy. If you are embarrassed about the shape you're in, you don't have to worry about anybody looking at you.

Your home workout will be very similar to the gym workout, since free weights are stressed in both systems.

With each exercise, a variation is suggested. Please do not try any of the variations until you have been working out for at least three months. Use the workout summary sheet provided at the end of the chapter once you have learned your routine and no longer need the instructions. It will serve as a quick reminder for you so that you don't inadvertently leave out an exercise or two.

PURCHASING HOME GYM EQUIPMENT

You will need the following:

- A set of each of the following dumbbells: 5's, 10's, 12's, 15's, 20's, and 25's.
- A barbell set with assorted weights.
- Ankle weights with slots for adding weights: 1's, 1½'s, 2's, 2½'s, and 5's.
- A padded exercise bench that adjusts to an incline.
- a 6-to-8-inch block of wood to place under the bench for decline exercises.

You can purchase your home gym equipment by consulting the following sources:

- *Muscle and Fitness* or *Shape* magazines. (Published by Joe Weider.)
- Triangle Health and Fitness Manufacturing (1-800-466-4111).
- Dan Lurie (718-978-4200). (Both Triangle and Dan Lurie will send you a free catalog, or will order for you without a catalog if you tell them over the phone what you want.)
- Department stores, such as *Sears, Roebuck; Herman's*, etc.
- Classified newspaper advertisements. People often sell home gym equipment at very reasonable prices.

Before starting your home workout, we think you should prepare yourself ahead of time for the possible distractions and arm yourself against them.

ADVANCE WARNING AGAINST DISTRACTIONS AT HOME

- The telephone. Unplug it or remove it from your workout area.
- Family members. Make sure they know that as far as they are concerned, when you are working out, you are "not home." Period.
- The door. Don't answer it. Remember. You're not home.

- The television, the refrigerator, the unfinished novel, the bed. Get your work-out out of the way. Then you can play. Remember: discipline, discipline, discipline. You are important. You deserve a beautiful body.
- Depression. Because no one is there to spur you on, you may find yourself being distracted by ennui, the feeling of indifference and what's-it-all-about. Fight that feeling. Your hard work will soon pay off.

CHEST ROUTINE

FLAT BENCH PRESS—CHEST EXERCISE #1

Follow the instructions on page 38.

CROSS BENCH PULLOVER—CHEST EXERCISE #2

DEVELOPS, SHAPES, TONES:
- Pectoral (chest) muscles.
- Serratus (side) muscles (minimal).
- Latissimus dorsi (minimal).

GET READY:
- Grasp a dumbbell in both hands. Place your palms against the inside plate and touch your thumbs together.
- Lie on a flat exercise bench. Place head at the end of the bench. Bend your knees.
- Raise your arms up so that the dumbbell is held above your upper chest area.

ACTION:
- Lower the dumbbell behind you until your arms are completely extended.
- Feel a full stretch in your pectoral area.
- Flex your chest as you raise the dumbbell to start position.
- Repeat the movement until you have completed your set.

CAREFUL:
- Control the dumbbell at all times. Don't thrust it up and let it drop down.
- Keep your mind on your chest. Don't let your arms do the work. Continually stretch and flex your chest muscles.

FOR A CHANGE:
- You can do this exercise with a barbell.

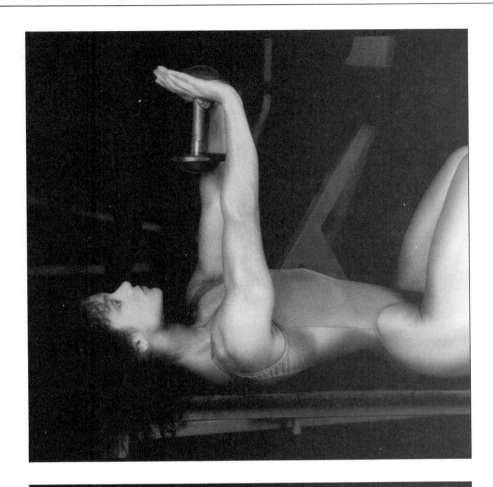

CROSS BENCH PULLOVER (START)

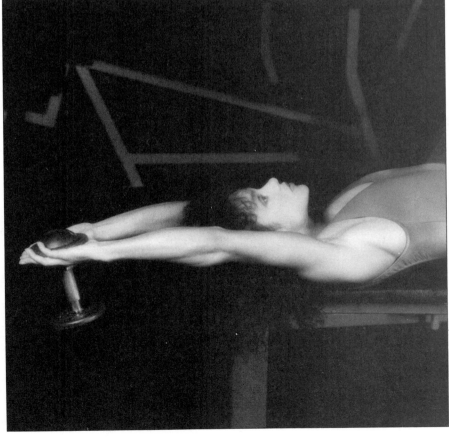

CROSS BENCH PULLOVER (FINISH)

SHOULDER ROUTINE

MILITARY PRESS TO THE REAR—SHOULDER EXERCISE #1

Follow the instructions on page 42.

SIDE LATERAL RAISE—SHOULDER EXERCISE #2

Follow the instructions on page 44.

BACK ROUTINE

ONE-ARM DUMBBELL BENT ROW—BACK EXERCISE #1

DEVELOPS, SHAPES, TONES:	• Upper and middle back area. • Latissimus dorsi—lats—which give the back a lean "V" look.
GET READY:	• Kneel with your left leg on a flat exercise bench. Keep your right leg straight. • Grasp a dumbbell in your right hand and let the dumbbell pull your arm straight down. • Keep your arm in direct line with your shoulder joint.
ACTION:	• Raise the dumbbell to your waist and flex your back as the dumbbell reaches its highest position. • Return to start and let the dumbbell stretch your back on the lowest position. • Repeat the movement until you have completed your set. • Repeat the set for the other arm.
CAREFUL:	• Never lose control of the weight and let it drop to start position. Don't jerk the weight up. • Keep your mind on your back muscles. Your arms should *not* be doing the work. • Be sure that you keep your starting position intact.
FOR A CHANGE:	• You can do a *barbell* bent row by standing in a slightly bent position and raising and lowering a barbell to your waist area. You will not need a bench.

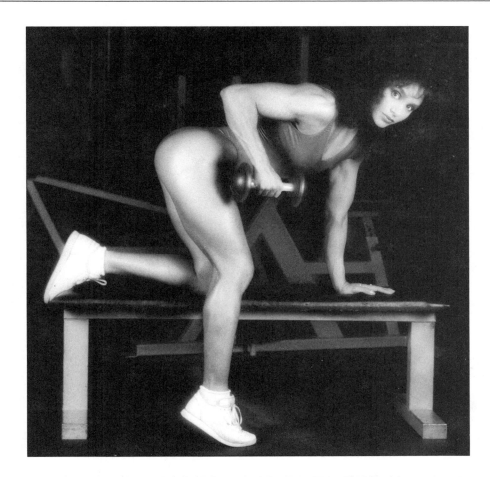

ONE-ARM DUMBBELL
BENT ROW (START)

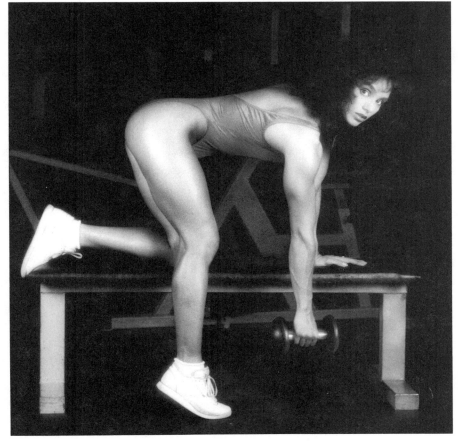

ONE-ARM DUMBBELL
BENT ROW (FINISH)

BENT-KNEE DEAD-LIFT—BACK EXERCISE #2

DEVELOPS, SHAPES, TONES:

- Upper back muscles.
- Latissimus dorsi (lats).
- Trapezius muscles (traps).

GET READY:

- Place a barbell in front of you, on the floor.
- Stand with feet a natural width apart.
- Hold the barbell a few inches wider than shoulder width.
- Bend your knees, squat, and look straight ahead.

ACTION:

- Rise to a standing position, keeping your head up and your back straight.
- Without resting, raise your shoulders up and back, as if you were shrugging your shoulders. Feel your upper back, latissimus dorsi, and trapezius muscles working.
- Be sure that your arms are straight down and that your elbows are locked as you shrug. The barbell should be resting against your thighs.
- Repeat the movement until you have completed your set.

CAREFUL:

- Be sure to stretch your back on the down movement and to flex your back on the up movement (as you shrug).
- Do not let your arms do the work. Keep your mind on your back.

FOR A CHANGE:

- You may do this exercise standing on a 6-inch wooden platform so that you can get a fuller stretch in the down position.

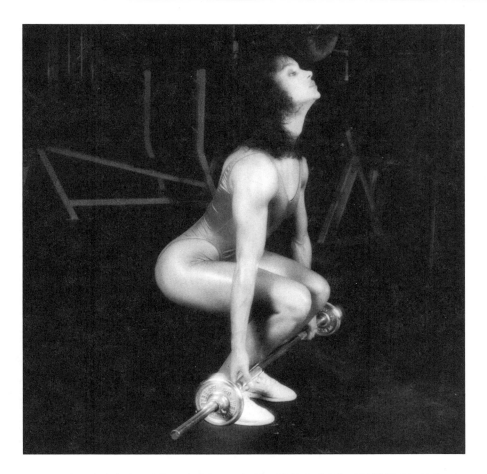

BENT-KNEE DEAD-LIFT (START)

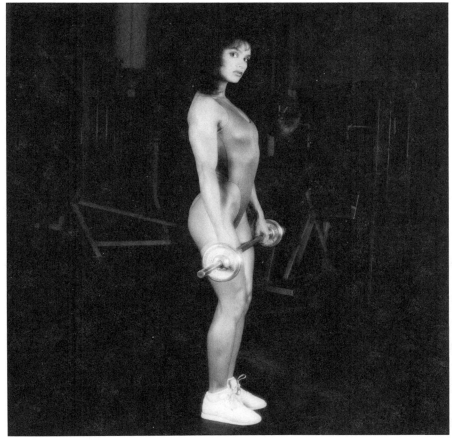

BENT-KNEE DEAD-LIFT (FINISH)

BICEPS ROUTINE

SEATED ALTERNATE BICEPS CURL—BICEPS EXERCISE #1
Follow the instructions on page 50.

CONCENTRATION CURL—BICEPS EXERCISE #2
Follow the instructions on page 52.

TRICEPS ROUTINE

DUMBBELL KICKBACK—TRICEPS EXERCISE #1

DEVELOPS, SHAPES, TONES:	• The entire triceps area.
GET READY:	• Lean against an exercise bench with your right hand as you place your bent right leg on the bench. • Hold a dumbbell in your left hand. • Keep your left elbow close to your waist area. Keep your left leg straight. Hold the dumbbell, palms facing body.
ACTION:	• Keep your elbow close to your body and extend your arm out behind you. • Return to start position and repeat the movement until you have completed your set. • Repeat the set for your other arm.
CAREFUL:	• Never let your elbow leave your waist. Keep it pinned. • Keep your mind on your triceps area. Watch and feel your triceps work. • You will not be able to use a heavy dumbbell for this very refined movement. Strict form is crucial.
FOR A CHANGE:	• You may do this exercise without the aid of a bench. Bend over and keep your arm pinned to your waist. Watch yourself perform the movement in the mirror.

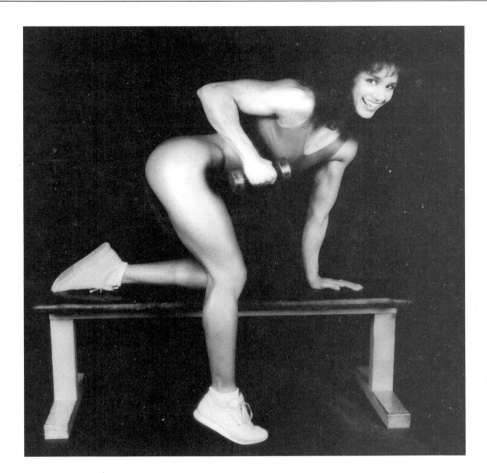

DUMBBELL KICKBACK (START)

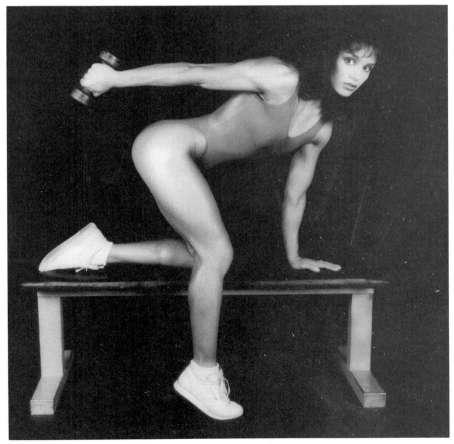

DUMBBELL KICKBACK (FINISH)

ONE-ARM TRICEPS EXTENSION—TRICEPS EXERCISE #2
Follow instructions on page 56.

L E G   R O U T I N E

LUNGE—LEG EXERCISE #1

DEVELOPS, SHAPES, TONES:
- Front quadriceps (thigh) muscle.
- Gluteus maximus (buttocks).
- Hips. Don't worry. It makes your butt and hips smaller, not larger. The word *develops* means "tightens" in this case.

GET READY:
- Place a barbell across your shoulders. Rest it on your trapezius muscles.
- Stand with your feet a natural width apart.
- Point your toes and keep feet in line with your knees. Keep them that way throughout the exercise.

ACTION:
- Step forward with your right foot. Bend your knee. Keep your torso from leaning forward. Look straight ahead in the mirror.
- Lunge as deeply as possible. Your alternate knee should nearly graze the floor.
- Without bouncing, return to start position and repeat the movement for your other leg.
- Repeat the movement for each leg until you have completed your set.

CAREFUL:
- Stretch your quadriceps muscle as you lunge.
- It will take time to get your balance for this exercise. You may feel uncoordinated for a month.
- Avoid the temptation to bounce off your leg while alternating legs. Control the movement.

FOR A CHANGE:
- Do this exercise on a block of wood (about 4 to 6 inches high). It will give you a fuller stretch in your quadriceps muscle.

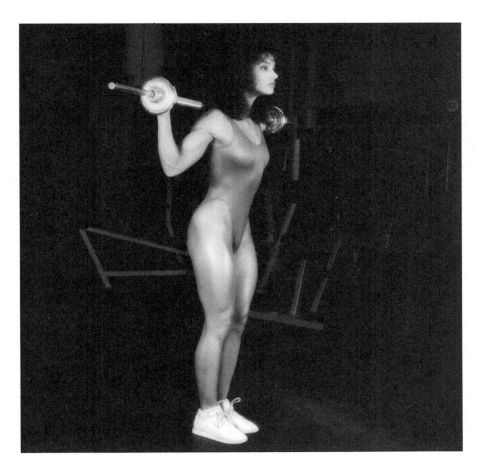

LUNGE (START)

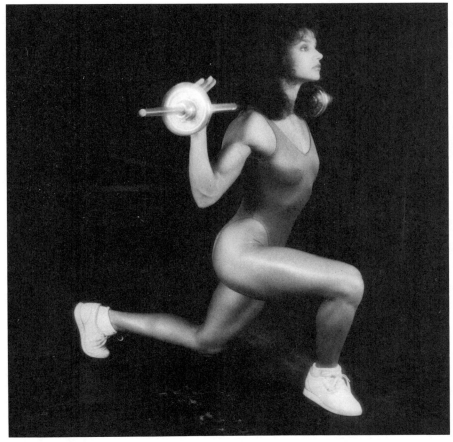

LUNGE (FINISH)

SQUAT—LEG EXERCISE #2

Follow instructions on page 60.

BUTTOCKS-HIP ROUTINE

FEATHER KICK-UP—BUTTOCKS-HIP EXERCISE #1

Follow the instructions on page 62.

BENCH SCISSORS—BUTTOCKS-HIP EXERCISE #2

Follow the instructions on page 64.

ABDOMINAL ROUTINE

SIT-UP—ABDOMINAL EXERCISE #1

Follow the instructions on page 66.

LEG RAISE—ABDOMINAL EXERCISE #2

Follow the instructions on page 68.

WORKOUT SUMMARY

Chest
1. Flat Bench Press
2. Cross Bench Pullover

Shoulder
1. Military Press to the Rear
2. Side Lateral Raise

Back
1. One-arm Dumbbell Bent Row
2. Bent-knee Dead-lift

Biceps
1. Seated Alternate Biceps Curl
2. Concentration Curl

Triceps
1. Dumbbell Kickback
2. One-arm Triceps Extension

Legs
1. Lunge
2. Squat

Buttocks-hip
1. Feather Kick-up
2. Bench Scissors

Abdominals
1. Sit-up
2. Leg Raise

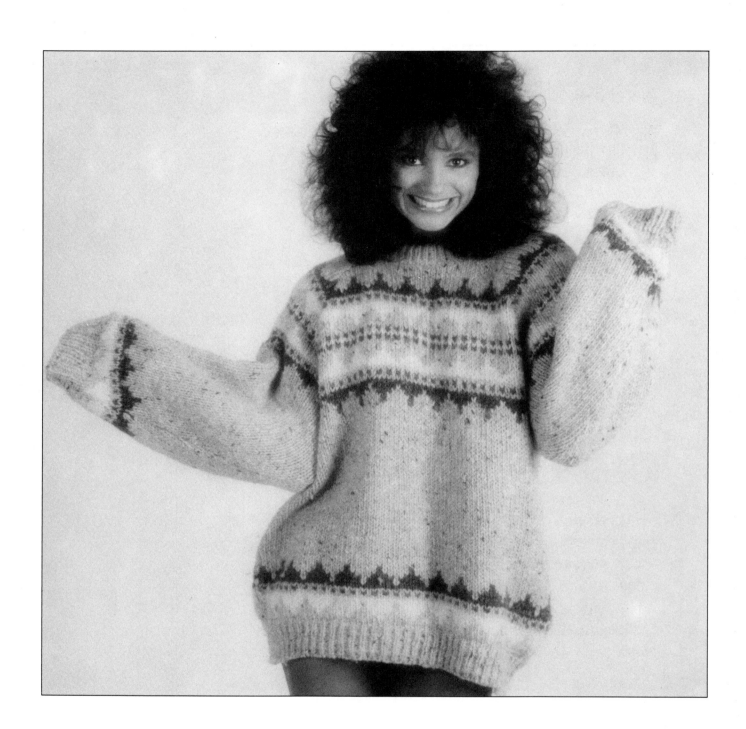

EXPRESS TRAINING PROBLEM AREAS

You may be anxious to see quick progress on one or two particular areas of your body. If you feel this way, you probably won't mind putting in an extra seven minutes per workout for that bodypart. All you have to do is check this chapter for the bodypart you want to "bomb" and add those exercises to your regular routine for that bodypart.

For example, if you want to speed up the progress on your buttocks-thigh area, in addition to doing your two required exercises (feather kick-up and bench scissors) you would add one or two additional exercises (the leg lift and/or the barbell tuck, listed next).

BUTTOCKS-HIP AREA

LEG LIFT WITH A WEIGHT—
BUTTOCKS-HIP EXPRESS EXERCISE #1

DEVELOPS, SHAPES, TONES:

- Buttocks (tightened and lifted).
- Back thigh (biceps femoris).
- Hip (narrowed and elongated).

GET READY:

- Place ankle weights or ankle bracelet and cable attachment on your ankles.
- Lean on a flat exercise bench with your right knee bent and your left leg extended straight down toward the floor.
- Stretch your foot back.

ACTION:

- Squeeze (flex) your buttocks. Lock your knee. Extend your left leg out behind you as high as possible. Be sure to keep your toes pointed back and your knee locked.
- Return to start position and repeat the movement until you have completed your set.
- Repeat the set for your right leg.
- Continue to alternate legs until you have performed 3 full sets. There is no rest between sets since each leg is getting a natural rest while the other is working.

CAREFUL:

- Do not jerk your leg up. Move quickly but control the weight.
- Continue to flex your buttocks throughout the exercise.
- Do not bend your knee. Keep your leg straight.
- Be sure that your leg remains close to your body. Do not let your leg wander outward.

FOR A CHANGE:

- If you work out in a gym, alternate by doing the exercise with ankle weights instead of the pulley cables.

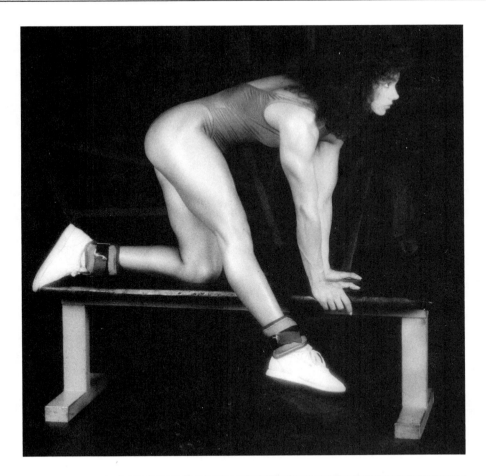

**LEG LIFT
WITH A WEIGHT (START)**

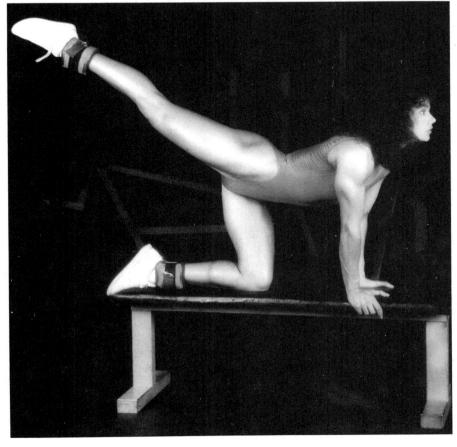

**LEG LIFT
WITH A WEIGHT (FINISH)**

BARBELL TUCK—BUTTOCKS-HIP EXPRESS EXERCISE #2

DEVELOPS, SHAPES, TONES:	• Entire buttocks area.
	• Upper hip area (smoothed and elongated).
GET READY:	• Place a light (25–45 pounds) barbell on your shoulder and stand with your feet a comfortable width apart. Be sure the barbell is resting on your trapezius muscles.
	• Perform the exercise in front of a mirror.
ACTION:	• Bend your knees and lower your body about 10 inches.
	• Flex your buttocks as hard as possible and begin to raise yourself to start position.
	• When you reach the highest point (start position), thrust your pelvic area forward and give it an extra hard flex.
	• Hold this tuck position for a split second.
	• Repeat the movement until you have completed your set.
CAREFUL:	• This entire exercise depends upon your diligence in flexing your buttocks area. Don't get lazy or let your mind wander.
	• Don't use a heavy barbell. The barbell is used only as an anchor for you.
FOR A CHANGE:	• You may do this exercise without a barbell if you are traveling and there is no barbell available. It works almost as well if you concentrate on the flexing.

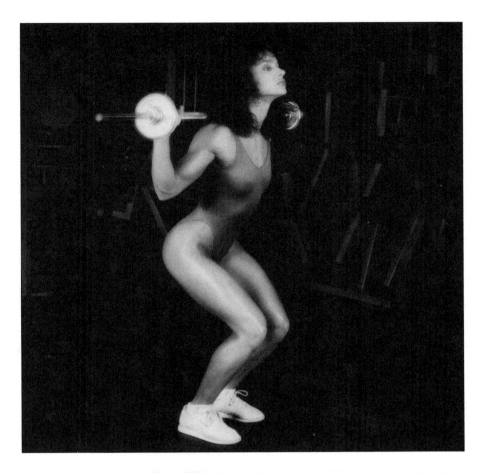

BARBELL TUCK (START)

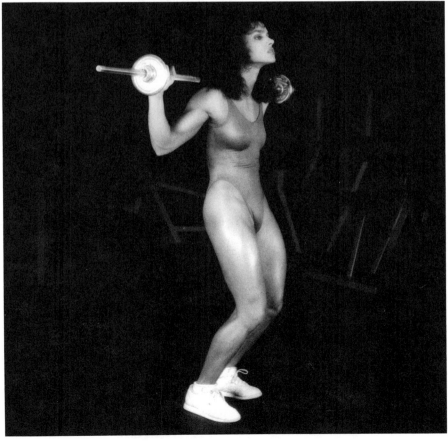

BARBELL TUCK (FINISH)

LEG AREA:

LEG CURL—EXPRESS LEG EXERCISE #1

DEVELOPS, SHAPES, TONES:
- Back thigh muscle (biceps femoris).

GET READY:
- Lie on the padded surface of a leg-curl machine, facedown, place your heels under the roller pads, and hold on to the sides of the bench.
- If you are performing this exercise without the machine, use ankle weights and lie, facedown, on a flat exercise bench.

ACTION:
- Bend your legs at the knees until they are perpendicular to your body.
- Hold the position for a split second and return to start.
- Repeat the movement until you have completed your set.

CAREFUL:
- Keep your mind on your back thighs (biceps femoris) as you perform the movement.
- Do not let the weight drop down quickly to start position. Control the weight at all times.
- Never jerk the weight up in an effort to avoid work.
- Keep your abdominal-hip area pressed to the bench throughout the exercise.

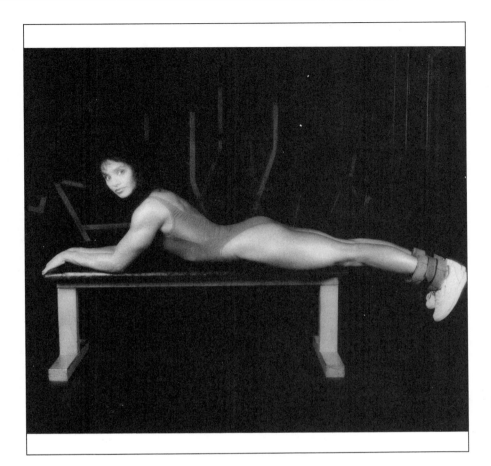

LEG CURL (START)

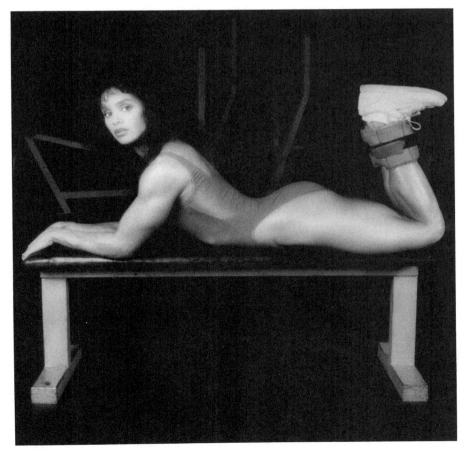

LEG CURL (FINISH)

PLIÉ SQUAT—EXPRESS LEG EXERCISE #2

DEVELOPS, SHAPES, TONES:

- Inner thigh
- Front thigh (quadriceps)
- Entire thigh area

GET READY:

- Grasp a dumbbell with both hands, palms facing your body.
- Hold the dumbbell in the center of your body, arms extended straight down and elbows nearly locked.
- Place your feet about 3 inches wider than shoulder width apart and point your toes outward. Be sure that your toes are in line with your knees.

ACTION:

- Lower your body to a squat position by slowly descending until you have reached an approximate 45 percent angle.
- Return to start position, keeping your back erect and your knees in line with your toes. Flex (squeeze) your front and inner thigh muscles as you reach start position.
- Without resting, repeat the movement until you have completed your set.

CAREFUL:

- Never arch your back or allow your buttocks to extend out behind you during this exercise. Keep your back straight as you perform the movement.
- Do not bend your elbows during the exercise. Remember that the weight is to serve as an anchor to be resisted by your working legs. Your arms should never move the weight.
- Don't forget to flex your entire thigh muscle on the up position of each repetition.

FOR A CHANGE:

- Do this exercise with a barbell. It may take time to learn to grip the barbell so that it remains balanced throughout the movement.

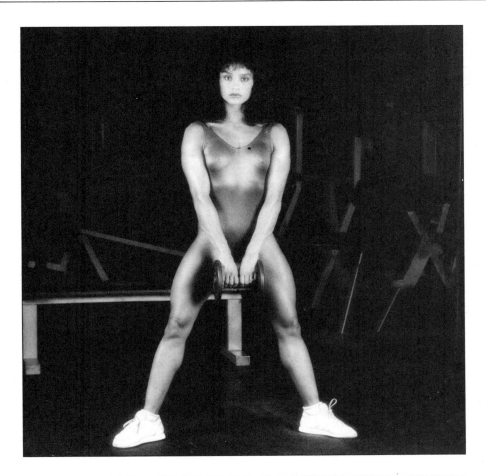

PLIÉ SQUAT (START)

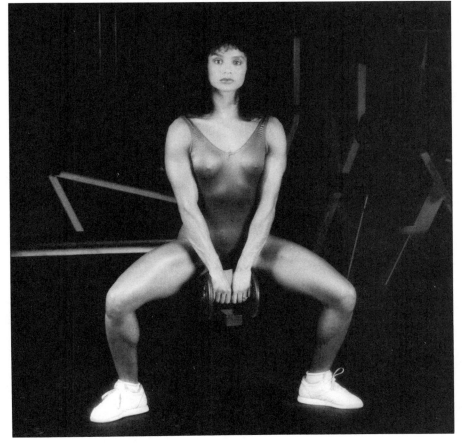

ALTERNATING BICEPS CURL
PLIÉ SQUAT (FINISH)

A B D O M I N A L   A R E A

LEG-IN WITH A WEIGHT—EXPRESS ABDOMINAL EXERCISE #1

DEVELOPS, SHAPES, TONES:	• Lower abdominal area.
GET READY:	• Wearing ankle weights, sit on a flat exercise bench. Place your buttocks close to the edge of the bench.
	• Lean back slightly and grasp the sides of the bench.
	• Extend your legs straight out in front of you.
ACTION:	• Bring your knees in until they are nearly touching your face.
	• Return to start position and repeat the movement until you have completed your set.
CAREFUL:	• Don't rush through the exercise. Keep your lower abdominal muscles flexed at all times.
	• Don't hold your breath. Breathe naturally.
FOR A CHANGE:	• You may perform this exercise by attaching a machine pulley to ankle bracelets or a two-footed strap (ask your gym owner if he or she has them).

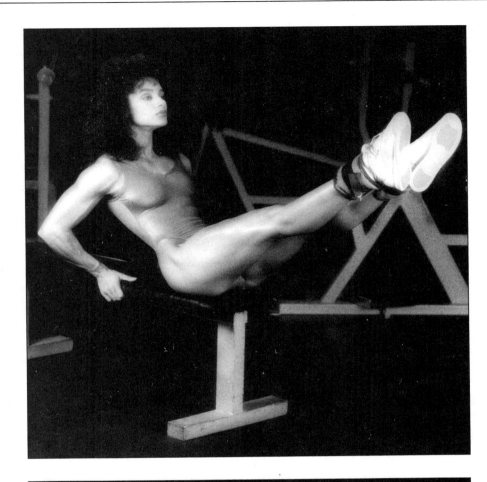

**LEG-IN WITH A WEIGHT
(START)**

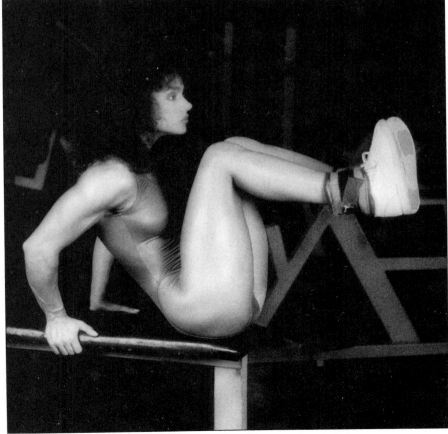

**LEG-IN WITH A WEIGHT
(FINISH)**

CRUNCH—EXPRESS ABDOMINAL EXERCISE #2

DEVELOPS, SHAPES, TONES:	• Upper abdominal area.
GET READY:	• Lie on the floor, flat on your back, and cross your legs at the ankles. • Place your hands, folded, behind your neck.
ACTION:	• Curl your body upward until your shoulders are lifted off the floor. Be sure that your abdominal muscles are doing the lifting work. • Return to start position and without resting even for a split second, repeat the movement until you have completed your set.
CAREFUL:	• Lift only your shoulders, not your back. • Keep your abdominal muscles flexed throughout the exercise. • Throw your mind into your abdominals and picture them taking shape as you exercise. • Do not lurch off the floor or nearly drop to start position. Control your movement. • Do not hold your breath. Breathe naturally.
FOR A CHANGE:	• You may place your legs over a flat exercise bench for support.

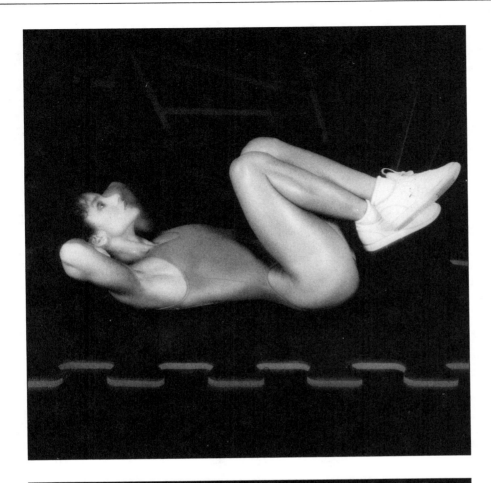

CRUNCH (START)

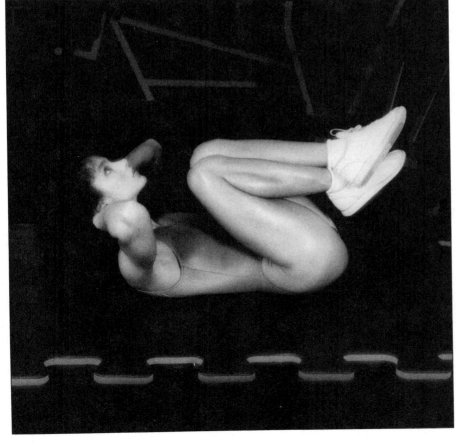

CRUNCH (FINISH)

TRICEPS AREA

CLOSE GRIP BENCH PRESS—EXPRESS TRICEPS EXERCISE #1

DEVELOPS, SHAPES, TONES:
- The entire triceps area.

GET READY:
- Lie on a flat exercise bench.
- Grip the barbell. Place your hands about 8 inches apart. Face your palms upward.

ACTION:
- Raise the barbell until your arms are completely extended and your elbows locked.
- Lower the barbell until it nearly grazes the center of your pectoral area.
- Keep your mind on your triceps area. This is *not* a chest exercise. The bench press, you will recall, is done with a much wider grip.
- Be sure to stretch your triceps on the downward movement and to flex your triceps on the upward movement.

CAREFUL:
- Never widen your grip to more than 10 inches apart (thumb to thumb).
- Never jerk the weight up or let it drop down too quickly.
- Don't try to use too heavy a weight. This is a tricky movement and requires delicate muscular manipulation. Do the exercise in strict form, and use weights as light as necessary.

FOR A CHANGE:
- You can vary your grip, making it as narrow as 6 inches thumb to thumb and going the full range to 10 inches from thumb to thumb for a week or two at a time.

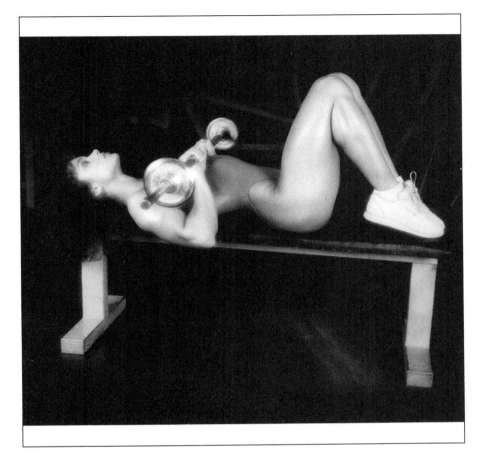

CLOSE GRIP BENCH PRESS
(START)

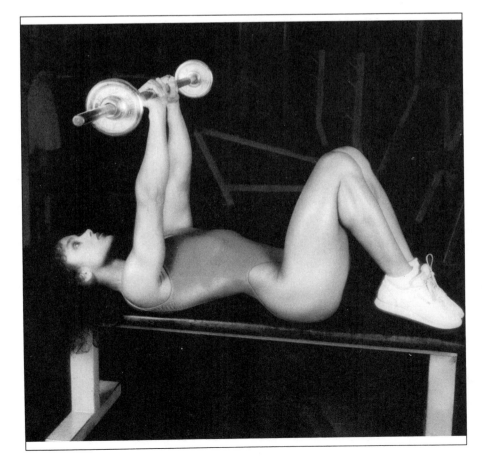

CLOSE GRIP BENCH PRESS
(FINISH)

DIPS BETWEEN BENCHES—EXPRESS TRICEPS EXERCISE #2

DEVELOPS, SHAPES, TONES:	• The entire triceps area, especially the upper triceps area, which presents the most problem to the majority of women. This exercise is very difficult at first, but well worth the breaking-in period. Do not give up. You will get it. It takes time.
GET READY:	• Line up two flat exercise benches so that they are parallel to each other and wide enough apart to support you when you lean on one with the palms of your hands and on the other with the heels of your feet. (You may pile up blocks of wood if another bench is not available.)
	• Place your hands behind you about 8 inches apart and grip the bench as you curl your fingers around the edge of the bench.
ACTION:	• In full control, lower your body as far as possible by letting your upper arms bend fully. Your triceps will stretch out on the downward movement.
	• Raise yourself by straightening your arms fully. Feel your triceps doing the work. Flex your triceps on the top position and repeat the movement until you have completed your set.
	• You will do 3 sets of 15 repetitions (after a few months—at first you will be lucky to get 3 sets of 3 repetitions). Eventually you will place a dumbbell on your lap, graduating the weight of the dumbbell for each set so that you will be pyramiding the weight just as you do for other exercises. At that time you will do 12–15 reps for your first set, 8–10 reps for your second set, and 6–8 reps for your last set. This may take a few months, but eventually you will do it with ease and laugh when you remember the initial struggle.
CAREFUL:	• Do not lurch to the upward position or drop quickly to the down position. Control the movement and throw your mind into the triceps muscles. Picture your triceps becoming tight and strong.
FOR A CHANGE:	• Vary your grip between 4 and 10 inches.

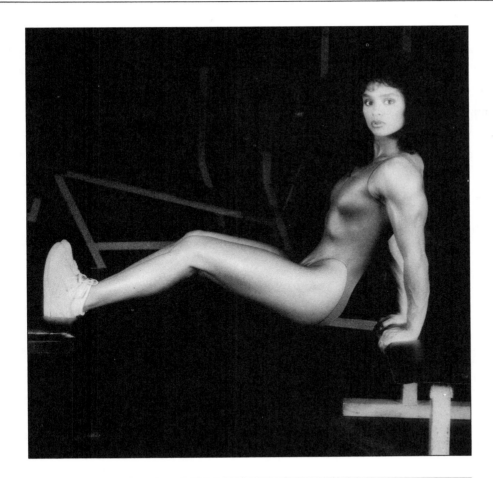

**DIPS BETWEEN BENCHES
(START)**

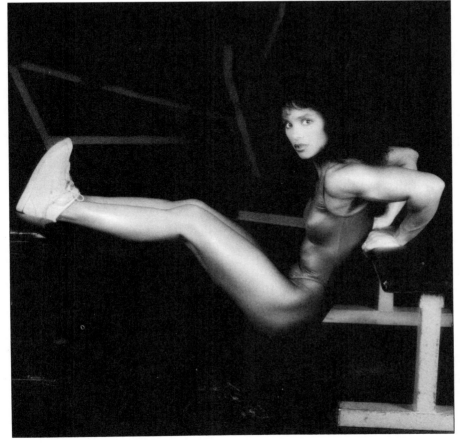

**DIPS BETWEEN BENCHES
(FINISH)**

In addition to "bombing" problem areas, you may want to speed up your general progress by using some express methods on your entire body.

SPEEDING UP THE PROGRESS ON YOUR ENTIRE BODY:

1. Add an additional set to each of your regular exercises. Do set 1 at 15 repetitions, then:

   Set 2 at 12 reps
   Set 3 at 10 reps
   Set 4 at 6–8 reps

2. Do one extra exercise for each bodypart. Select one of the "For a change" exercises listed for each exercise. For example, if you wish to speed up the progress on everything, and you are starting with your chest, you may choose to do the incline bench press listed in the "For a change" section of the flat bench press exercise.

3. Do two extra exercises for each bodypart. Do the suggested "For a change" variations in addition to the required exercise, and the "express" exercises.

4. Work out an additional day. Instead of a 2-day-a-week workout, do a 3-day-a-week workout, but remember, never two days in a row.

In order to speed up your progress overall, you may want to use some of the following special fat-burning techniques.

1. Do three 20-minute aerobic sessions per week. You may run or walk (if you walk, you must walk double the running time, 40 minutes to equal the 20-minute run.), ride the stationary bicycle, jump rope, jump on the trampoline, or swim.

2. Do up to five 30-minute aerobic sessions (never, ever, more, no matter how desperate you are. You will only burn away precious muscle).

3. Superset. Combine both exercises for a bodypart. For example, for the chest routine, do set 1 of your bench press at 15 repetitions, and then, without resting, do your first set of 15 repetitions of your other chest exercise, the incline flye. Then, without resting, do your second set of the bench press with a higher weight at 10 repetitions and quickly proceed to your incline flye with the 10 repetitions, and so on. You will not rest at all,

but, of course, just walking from one station to the next and getting into position will provide a "survival" rest.

Note: This "superset" method helps to provide an aerobic fat-burning effect. It also helps you to get through your workout more quickly. But be careful. Don't get sloppy and start to cut the movement short. Be strict or you will defeat your purpose.

HOW MANY EXPRESS TECHNIQUES SHOULD YOU USE AT ONCE?

You may use one or two of the techniques, or you may use all of them. Chances are, you will find yourself experimenting with one and then another. We suggest that you try two for a few months. Then drop those two and try another two until you have tried them all. Then you can decide which ones you may want to keep as a regular part of your routine.

WHAT IF I DON'T USE THE EXPRESS METHODS? HOW LONG WILL IT TAKE ME TO GET INTO SHAPE?

Each express method will increase your progress by at least one-fourth. If you use two or three methods, you may double your progress. But we are not at all concerned with time. We have discovered that patience is the key to achieving lasting results. So if you do not have the time or energy to use the express techniques, don't be discouraged. You will get to your goal of a perfectly formed hard body, only it will take a little longer. But you *will* get there.

STICKING POINTS

You may find that after having made some progress on a given bodypart, suddenly your progress seems to stagnate—nothing appears to be happening. Don't get discouraged. The body hits "plateaus" and stays visibly the same from time to time. This is a normal part of the growth process. When it happens, continue to train hard and to envision your body the way you want it to look. Realize that suddenly, one day, you will be looking in the mirror and to your surprise you will notice a visible improvement in that bodypart. Thirty-two-year-old Candy says: "I was working my buttocks so hard that I thought for sure I would see a big change in a month, but nothing happened. I was so depressed I thought that maybe the whole program was a waste of time. Then I just didn't look back there for a while and when I did, after another two months, wow, was I surprised. It just seems to happen overnight—once it happens."

So, no matter how discouraged you may feel, make this your motto: *Keep going.* Continue to train, and in time you will see results. That's a promise.

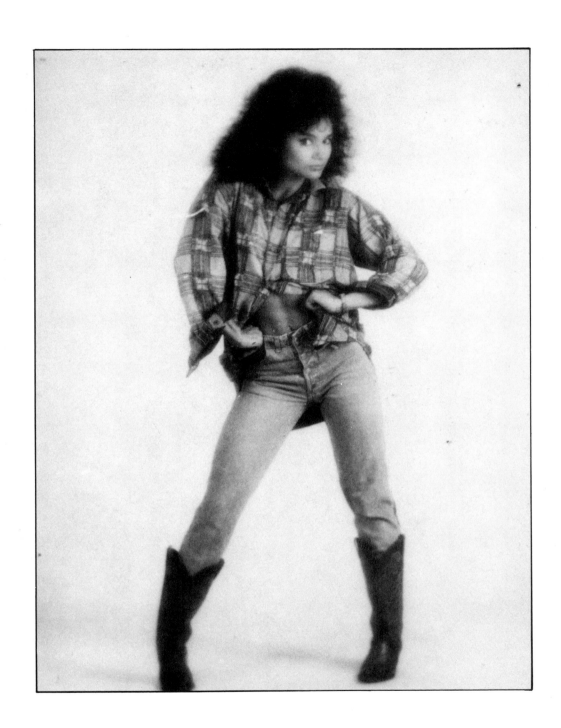

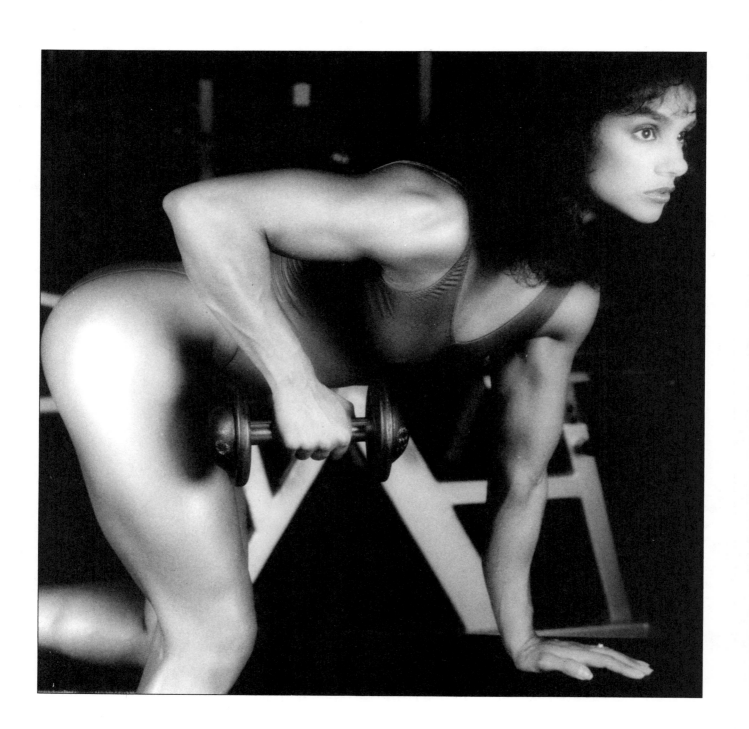

EATING STRATEGIES FOR WOMEN ON THE RUN

It is possible for you to eat delicious, nutritious food even though you are very busy and have little time to spare. There's no reason to believe that just because you don't have time to cook elaborate meals or sit down to leisurely lunches or dinners, you must sacrifice good eating. In reality, the best foods are the ones that are most easily prepared. For example, how much time does it take to wash and scrape a raw carrot?

Most people "get fat" because of haphazard eating. Your body responds to high-calorie eating by storing the excess calories as fat, about one pound of fat for every 3,500 excess calories you consume. This storage system is part of the innate survival mechanism of the body. The body saves up excess fat for a possible future famine. Your goal is to eliminate excess calories so that unattractive fat will not be stored on your body.

Although *this* eating program will not require you to count calories, it is important that you have a basic idea of how calories work to keep you lean or make you fat.

THE FUNCTION OF CALORIES

A calorie is a unit of energy supplied to your body when you eat food, so that your body can function and stay alive. You need calories supplied by food even to breathe and to sleep (you burn about 40 calories an hour sleeping). As you know, people who are unable to eat are fed intravenously so that their bodily functions will continue to perform. Thus, a calorie is not an enemy. Too many calories, however, are an enemy. For this reason it is important to avoid foods that are not nutritious yet are high in calories. These foods will be discussed later along with low-calorie foods that are nutritious.

WHAT THE BODY NEEDS

To function correctly, the body needs a balance of carbohydrates, protein, and fat, and a proper supply of essential vitamins, minerals, and water.

CARBOHYDRATES

Carbohydrates supply the body with its main source of energy. They are digested and broken down into glucose, or "blood sugar," which is what keeps the brain and central nervous system functioning. If your diet is lacking in carbohydrates, protein, which is the tissue-building substance of your diet, will not be used to build tissue but will instead be used up as energy to replace your carbohydrate deficit. So an inadequate carbohydrate supply can hinder muscle growth.

About two-thirds of your calories should come from carbohydrates, the other third should come from protein and fat.

PROTEIN

Protein is the basic building material of the body. Muscles, hair, nails, blood, and internal organs are made up of protein. Protein also affects water balance and metabolism.

Protein is made up of twenty-two elements called "amino acids." Since the human body cannot produce eight of these amino acids, it is essential that we eat foods that contain them. One can find them in such foods as fish, poultry, red meat, milk and milk products, and eggs. Combinations of such foods as rice and beans can provide the essential amino acids for people who are vegetarians and cannot otherwise obtain them from other sources of protein such as fish.

Protein should comprise about one-sixth of your calories, or about 16⅓ percent.

FAT

Although most of us consume too much fat, a minimum amount is necessary for good health. Without fat, vitamins A, E, K, and D as well as the mineral calcium could not be absorbed by the body. Fat also provides a cushion for the internal organs as well as a cushion under your skin. When too much fat builds up under the skin, however, the cushion becomes too thick and obscures shapely muscle.

CHOLESTEROL

Cholesterol is hard or solid fat and is found in red meats, eggs, cheese, and butter. Cholesterol, in excess, causes arteriosclerosis, heart attacks, and other illnesses, but in moderate amounts it is essential to your diet. Sunlight converts cholesterol into vitamin D, which aids in the digestion of carbohydrates. Cholesterol helps form cortisone and sex hormones, so a moderate amount is important for good health.

Your diet should comprise about one-sixth, or 16⅓ percent fat. If you keep your fat level this low (the average American consumes about 35 percent to 40 percent fat), you will never have to worry about high cholesterol.

VITAMINS

Vitamins are organic substances necessary for growth, vitality, general well-being, and the maintenance of life itself. The best sources of vitamins are fresh or frozen foods. Supplements can be taken but should never be used as a substitute for good eating. Only after you consult your doctor should anything more than a multivitamin be taken. If you eat plenty of the delicious energy-yielding foods mentioned in this chapter, there should be no need for supplements.

MINERALS

Minerals are nutrients found in organic and inorganic combinations. Bones, teeth, soft tissue, muscle, blood, and nerve cells are made up of minerals. Minerals are necessary for strong bones and a healthy heart. They help to keep the brain and nervous system functioning properly, and play a role in balancing the water content of the body.

HOW TO GET THE PROPER COMBINATION OF CARBOHYDRATES, PROTEINS, FATS, VITAMINS, AND MINERALS

Your daily food intake should comprise two-thirds carbohydrates, one-sixth protein, and one-sixth fat. Choose your foods from the carbohydrate, protein, and vitamin and mineral charts in this chapter.

GOOD SOURCES OF CARBOHYDRATES

There are three sources of carbohydrates: processed, simple, and complex. The processed ones are the bad guys, such as sugar in every form. We will not, of course, include any of them in our "good" list. Legitimate carbohydrates fall into two categories: simple and complex. Simple carbohydrates are fruits. You can use them when you want an immediate source of energy. Complex carbohydrates provide you with a gradually released source of energy. They are found in vegetables, rice, and grains.

Choose any foods from the following lists for your daily carbohydrate consumption.

Note: The foods followed by an * are higher in calories, so avoid them if you are trying to keep your calories very low in order to lose weight (fat).

SIMPLE CARBOHYDRATES FOR IMMEDIATE ENERGY

apples	oranges
apricots*	peaches
bananas*	pears
blackberries	persimmons
blueberries	pineapple
boysenberries	plantains*
cantaloupe	plums
cherries*	pomegranates*
cranberries*	prunes*

currants*	raisins*
dates*	raspberries
figs*	rhubarb
grapefruit	strawberries
grapes*	tangerines
nectarines	watermelon

COMPLEX CARBOHYDRATES FOR GRADUALLY RELEASED ENERGY

BREADS, FLOURS, CEREALS, GRAINS, AND GRAIN PRODUCTS

bran products: muffins, cereal, raw bran
buckwheat cereal
cornbread or corn muffins*
granola (without added sugar)*
pasta: high-protein or whole wheat
pumpernickel bread*
rice: brown or white
rye bread*
wheat germ
whole wheat products: pita bread, regular bread, cereals, etc.

VEGETABLES

alfalfa sprouts	chard
artichokes*	chives
asparagus	collards
bamboo shoots	corn*
beans: lentil,* lima,* kidney,* soy,* pinto*	cucumber
beans: green, yellow	dandelion greens
beets*	eggplant
broccoli	endive
brussels sprouts	kale
cabbage	leeks
carrots	lettuce
cauliflower	mushrooms
celery	mustard greens

okra	shallots
onions	spinach
scallions	tomatoes
peppers (red, green)	turnips
potatoes	turnip greens
pumpkin*	water chestnuts
radish	watercress
rutabaga	yams*
sauerkraut	

You can make delicious food combinations using the above foods and combining them with the protein list. For example, you can have protein linguine and red clam sauce, all sorts of delicious fruit or vegetable-salad mixtures, various rice and potato dishes, fish, chicken, and beef stews, and so on. There are lots of calorie-conscious cookbooks on the market today to assist you in your creative endeavors. (See bibliography for *Supercut*.)

GOOD SOURCES OF PROTEINS

MEATS AND POULTRY

brains—all kinds*	kidney
chicken—dark meat*	lamb*
chicken—white meat	liver*
chuck roast*	porterhouse steak*
club steak*	sirloin steak*
flank steak*	turkey—dark meat*
ground beef*	turkey—white meat
heart	veal*

Always remove excess fat from beef, and skin from turkey or chicken.

FISH AND SEAFOOD

bass*	mackerel*
bluefish*	oysters*
carp*	perch
clams	pike*
codfish*	salmon*
crab	shrimp
flounder	snapper
haddock	swordfish*
halibut*	trout, rainbow*
herring*	tuna
lobster	whitefish*

Remember to buy only tuna in water. Rinse the tuna to eliminate excess sodium.

DAIRY PRODUCTS

low-fat, low-salt cottage cheese
low-fat mozzarella cheese*
grated or hard Parmesan cheese*
low-fat ricotta cheese*
eggs
low-fat milk
low-fat yogurt

GOOD SOURCES OF FAT

This may seem like a strange category. Who, after all, has to go out of her way to find fatty foods? There is plenty of fat in ice cream, fried foods, or fatty meats. But these are non-nutritious ways of fulfilling your fat allotment. The fact is, you don't have to go out of your way to get your fat at all. You'll find that by just eating your daily protein requirement, you've already used up your fat allowance. Why? All complete protein foods listed above have quite a few calories in fat. Foods, as you may know, do not consist of only one food component. Let's look at white-meat chicken and flounder, for example.

FOOD	CARBOHYDRATE *Calories*	PROTEIN *Calories*	FAT *Calories*	TOTAL *Calories*
6 oz. chicken breast	Zero	225	110	335
6 oz. flounder	Zero	150	50	200

Notice that although white-meat chicken and flounder are considered to be among the lowest in fat content, they still contain a certain amount of fat calories.

Most foods you eat contain some fat. Even the innocent apple, which is a good carbohydrate food and has only about 80 calories, consists of 70 carbohydrate calories and about 10 fat calories. It is obviously not necessary to eat such foods as butter, mayonnaise, ice cream, etc., which consist of almost 100 percent fat calories to fulfill the fat requirement.

GOOD SOURCES OF VITAMINS

You will notice that some foods are mentioned in many vitamin lists. This means it is a food that should be at the top of your regular shopping list, because it can serve your varied vitamin needs.

VITAMIN A

alfalfa	kale
broccoli	liver
carrots	spinach
eggs	yellow fruits and vegetables
fish	

VITAMIN B COMPLEX

organ meats	whole grains
wheat germ	yogurt

VITAMIN B-1

brown rice	organ meats
fish meat	poultry
lobster	wheat germ

VITAMIN B-2

eggs	organ meats
fruit	poultry
green leafy vegetables	whole grains

VITAMIN B-6

bananas	meat	wheat germ
cabbage	organ meats	whole grains
fish	prunes*	
green leafy vegetables	raisins*	

VITAMIN B-12

beef	milk and milk products
eggs	organ meats

NIACIN

breads and cereals	milk products	seafood
eggs	organ meats	whole grains
lean meats	poultry	

VITAMIN C

oranges and all fresh fruits and vegetables

VITAMIN D

beef liver	organ meats
egg yolks	sunlight

VITAMIN E

dark green vegetables	organ meats
eggs	wheat germ
fruits	

GOOD SOURCES OF MINERALS

CALCIUM

After the age of thirty, men and women alike begin to experience a slight thinning and weakening of the bones, unless they do some weight-bearing exercises to prevent the condition. In addition to exercise, it is important to eat proper foods that contain a good supply of calcium. The result of a severe lack of calcium is the condition of osteoporosis—weakened, shortened bones. Following are some excellent sources of calcium.

The recommended daily allowance of calcium suggested by the United States Government is 800 to 1,200 mg. However, doctors today generally agree that 1,500 mg is ideal for women, and the United States Government allows this extra amount in their supplementary suggestion, which is 1,000 to 2,000 mg.

Because calcium is so important to your diet, we list the source as well as the mg. Make these foods a regular part of your diet and you won't have to count mg.

FOODS CONTAINING 100 MG OF CALCIUM

1 oz. part-skim mozzarella cheese
1 cup skim milk
1 oz. Swiss cheese
8 oz. plain yogurt
4 oz. scallops
1 cup farina
10 okra pods
1 cup cooked soybeans
1 cup broccoli
⅔ cup Cream of Wheat cereal
1 cup collard greens
1 cup mustard greens
1 cup kale
4 oz. tofu (bean curd)
1 cup low-fat cottage cheese
1 cup buttermilk
1 cup navy beans

⅔ cup oatmeal
4 oz. shrimp
1 cup Chinese stir-fry vegetables
1 cup dandelion greens
1 cup turnip greens

If you are concerned that you are not getting your daily requirement of calcium from natural food sources, you can take a supplement, but be sure you don't go over the recommended daily allowance. Research is now beginning to indicate that too much can be as detrimental as too little.

IRON

dark green, leafy vegetables	oysters
eggs	poultry
fish	shellfish
lean meats	wheat germ
liver	whole grains
organ meats	

MAGNESIUM

bran	organ meats	spinach
brown rice	seafood	
green vegetables	seaweed	

PHOSPHORUS

eggs	poultry
fish	seaweed
grains	yellow cheeses
meat	yogurt

POTASSIUM

apricots	figs*	red meats
bananas	lima beans*	seafood
broccoli	peaches	spinach
brussels sprouts	raisins*	yellow vegetables
dates*		

SODIUM

Although sodium is a needed mineral, most people consume much more than the recommended daily sodium allowance of 1,100–3,300 mg. For this reason we treat it as a "food enemy" (see following paragraphs). Typical natural sources of sodium are:

table salt
cheese
milk
seafood

CHOOSING A BALANCED DIET

Remember to choose two-thirds of your food from the carbohydrate group and one-third from the protein group. (You now know that the fat will automatically be included in the protein group so you don't have to go out of your way to eat fatty foods.)

Notice which foods occur again and again. Make those a regular part of your diet. Green leafy vegetables, yellow vegetables, organ meats, whole grains, and eggs appear on the lists of many of the categories.

WATER

Your internal organs are bathed by the pure water you drink. Water also moisturizes your skin. You should drink six to eight glasses a day. Water also helps to curb your appetite. Drink a glass before and after each meal, and you'll find that you've fulfilled your water requirement and curbed your appetite at the same time.

FOOD ENEMIES

Whether you are attempting to lose weight or maintain weight, it is a good idea to avoid the food enemies. They are: fat, sugar, and salt.

FAT

Red meats have an excess of fat, so you should keep them down to a minimum. Avoid all fried foods. Stay away from doughnuts, ice cream, pork, butter and margarine, and cream cheese. Check *The Nutrition Almanac* (see bibliography) for fat content, especially if you are trying to lose weight.

SUGAR

Processed sugars, such as are found in cakes, cookies, candies, and many breakfast cereals, give you a quick energy boost and then an immediate letdown that compels you to reach for more sweets. The result is the consumption of more non-nutritious or "empty" calories that are stored on your body as fat. Stay away from sugars and remember to read labels. Sugars are hidden behind such titles as: fructose, sucrose, and dextrose. Honey and molasses are also forms of non-nutritious sugar.

SALT

Salt, or sodium, holds up to fifty times its own weight in water. For this reason, someone who indulges in a high-sodium diet can appear ten pounds fatter than she really is. Excess sodium also causes high blood pressure. Avoid the following high-sodium foods: pickles, fast-food hamburgers and cheeseburgers, frankfurters, and all canned and smoked foods. Check food labels for sodium content. Never use table salt. Also, when eating in a Chinese restaurant, ask the waiter to serve your food without the MSG.

Where will you get your daily sodium requirement? From the foods you naturally eat. There is sodium in virtually everything. Tap water contains sodium. You get 600 mg of sodium in 6 ounces of flounder and 105 mg of sodium in 6 ounces of chicken breast. Even a cup of spinach has 50 mg of sodium, and would you believe it, half of a cantaloupe has 25 mg of sodium. A medium-size tomato has 4 mg of sodium and one cup of celery has 150 mg of sodium. You'll never have to worry about getting enough sodium in your diet.

SPICES

Learn to use spices in place of salt. Experiment with various combinations. Here are some hints:

Basil: Italian dishes, vegetables
Chives: eggs, seafood, fish
Dill: salads, cabbage, squash, fish
Marjoram: Italian dishes, chicken, lamb, eggs
Oregano: tomato sauces, chicken, eggplant, mushrooms

Rosemary: beets, cabbage, beef, lamb, or veal roast
Sage: cheeses, beef, all sorts of stews
Tarragon: vinaigrette dressing, veal, salmon
Thyme: beef, squash, onions, clams

LEMON AND VINEGAR

Experiment with lemon and vinegar. Add various spices to them and make salad dressings of different flavors. You can put lemon or vinegar on fish, chicken, beef—just about anything. Try putting wine vinegar on cottage cheese. It's delicious.

CAFFEINE

Too much caffeine can cause irritability and sleeplessness, although one or two cups of coffee are not harmful and can be a pleasant pickup. Be aware that most colas and chocolate drinks contain caffeine, so if you don't want to overindulge in caffeine, read labels and be careful.

ALCOHOL

Hard liquor and good health do not mix well. We recommend white wine or dry champagne rather than other, harsher, substances. You can have a glass or two of wine or champagne on the weekends and even during the week if you are at maintenance level. If you must drink hard liquor, do so only on rare occasions and when you do, avoid sweet mixes. Stick to club soda, water, orange juice, or grapefruit juice as mixers.

HOW TO LOSE WEIGHT

It takes a deficit of 3,500 calories to lose one pound of fat. If you want to lose weight, stick to the foods discussed above in balance, and temporarily avoid the ones marked with a *, because they are higher in calories. Completely avoid foods high in fat and sugar, and keep your sodium level low or you will gain water weight and feel and look fat.

REDUCE YOUR GENERAL CALORIC INTAKE.

You should limit your calorie intake to the range of 1,500 to 1,800 a day until you reach your weight goal. It is foolish to try to limit your calories to fewer than 1,500, because your body will rebel and the moment you go off the diet it will force you to eat more in preparation for the next famine time. If you eat 1,500 to 1,800 calories, your body will not think it is starving and will not lie in wait for an opportunity to gain it all back. Most diets fail because of drastic caloric drops. Be calm and lose the weight slowly, and it will surely stay off. An average of a pound a week of steady weight loss is perfect. If you lost a pound a week for a year, you'd be 52 pounds lighter next year, and you'd stay that way. There would be no "elevator" effect.

CREATE AN ENERGY DEFICIT.

Burn up more calories than you are consuming. By following this workout, you will be burning an additional 1,400 calories a week. You can do some additional exercises, such as three 20-minute sessions of aerobics: jump rope, ride a bicycle, run, swim, and so on. This will burn another 800 calories in a week. Between working out and the three 20-minute aerobic sessions, you will have burned up an extra 2,200 calories a week—over two-thirds of a pound of fat.

SPEED UP YOUR BASAL METABOLISM.

Your basal metabolism is the amount of energy your body uses to stay alive. Even if you were in a coma, your body would still burn energy to stay alive—to keep your heart beating, your blood circulating, and so on. The general definition of basal metabolism refers to the amount of energy your body uses when it is in a state of rest—sitting in a chair, for example, or sleeping.

You can increase your basal metabolism by putting muscle on your body, because muscle is the only body material that metabolizes or burns energy even in a state of rest. Once you put on muscle (after about three to six months of this program) your basal metabolism will increase so that whereas you previously burned, say, 40 calories an hour while sleeping or sitting in a chair, you will now burn about 60 calories an hour doing the same thing. Over a twenty-four-hour period you will have burned approximately an extra 480 calories that alone will keep a pound a week of fat off your body.

The speeding up of your basal metabolism because of the addition of muscle to your body is one of the most wonderful benefits that come to you as a result of working out with this program.

EAT MORE OFTEN.

Instead of eating one huge meal and two small meals or three big meals, eat three moderate-size meals and two good-size snacks or mini-meals. Suppose you are on a diet and wish to keep within a calorie range of 1,500 to 1,800 calories. Spread those calories out into ranges of, say: 400, 200, 400, 150, 350. The more often you eat, the more often your metabolism starts working hard to process and burn up the food being put into your body. Eating often works something like turning a car engine on and off frequently. The more you turn the car on and off, the more fuel you use. The more often you eat, the more often the engine of your body goes "on" and the more fuel (calories) is used. Eating lots of small meals is a much more efficient way to burn calories than starving all day long and eating all of the allotted calories in one huge meal at night. When this inefficient method of eating occurs, the metabolism slows down to a near halt during the day, so that instead of burning the normal, say, 60 calories an hour at rest you would burn 30 calories. The body's survival instinct tells the metabolism to slow down because no food is coming in. The body does not know how long this will last, so, to preserve energy, it slows down. That's why you feel an energy lull at a certain point when you haven't eaten in five or six hours.

By waiting so long to eat, you have defeated your purpose. You have burned, say, 300 calories less in the time you didn't eat. Had you eaten, you could have enjoyed the 300 calories, felt energetic, and burned them off more easily because of the turning-on-and-off-often effect—and what's more, you wouldn't have felt deprived and depressed.

HOW TO EAT ON THE RUN
IF YOU ARE ON A DIET

There are certain foods listed and not listed that can be consumed conveniently on the run. Here are some ideas:

Soft pretzels sold by street vendors (shake off excess salt)
A slice of pizza (blot off excess fat with a napkin)
a couple of pieces of fruit
a cup of yogurt
a small container of cottage cheese
an English muffin with a teaspoon of jelly
an order of whole wheat toast with a teaspoon of jelly
a bagel with a teaspoon of butter
a bowl of soup and crackers
a bran muffin

You may wonder how you can eat pizza (about 350 calories a slice when blotted) or a large soft pretzel (about 400 calories for a very large one). Why not? They are legitimate carbohydrates, even if not perfect carbohydrates, and they are appealing to the taste. True, the crust of the pizza and the soft pretzel are made with bleached flour, but eating such foods every so often will do you no harm at all, and you'll enjoy them.

A teaspoon of jelly isn't all that fattening (about 30 calories) and it may satisfy your sweet tooth. A pat of butter is only about 45 calories, and a bowl of soup, although usually high in sodium, won't harm you if you generally keep an eye on your sodium intake (eliminate all canned, smoked foods, etc.).

ORDERING FOOD IN A RESTAURANT

There are plenty of nonfattening foods that can be ordered when eating out:

chef's salad (avoid the ham and limit the beef; tell them to give you extra turkey instead.)
linguine and red clam sauce
Tuna in water with lemon wedges
tossed salad
cottage cheese
poached eggs and dry whole wheat toast
broiled fish or chicken
white-meat turkey sandwich on whole wheat
shrimp cocktail
clams on the half shell

steamed mussels
baked potato
white rice, no butter
diet soda, club soda, Perrier water
orange juice, grapefruit juice

And plenty more. The idea is to avoid fat, sugar, and excess salt.

HOW TO MAINTAIN YOUR WEIGHT: GOOD NEWS—YOU CAN INDULGE ONCE A WEEK.

Once you have achieved the happy body condition you want, you can maintain your weight by eating according to the above guidelines on a daily basis and eating whatever you please once a week. Select one day a week and "go to town." Have that ice-cream cone, that greasy hamburger, that box of candy— whatever. As long as you go right back to good eating habits the next day, you'll maintain your weight. You don't have to eat junk food on your free day, however. You may want to eat high-calorie good foods, and maybe larger portions of them. For example, you may decide to have some rich Italian dish composed of a cheesy, meaty sauce with pasta. The point is, you can enjoy life and still remain slim, once you get slim *if* you don't fall into the trap of binging every day.

Keep a watch on your food intake daily and you'll be free to indulge on birthdays, holidays, and the like. There may be occasions when you break your good eating for a few days at a time. If this is so, just cut your intake for a week or so after the vacation from good eating. Get back on an even keel before things get out of hand so that you won't have to diet for an extensive period of time.

But no matter what, remember that there is nothing to dread or fear in food. Food is wonderful, and even if you are dieting you can eat lots of healthful, appealing, nutritious foods. Never panic if you've gained a lot of weight and have to diet again. So what. It will come off just as systematically as it got on you. You didn't gain 30 pounds overnight. It may have seemed that way, but it took at least fifteen to twenty weeks. You can surely lose it in the same time. Just relax and do the right thing, and the excess pounds will come off.

OTHER EATING TIPS

DON'T EAT DIRECTLY BEFORE A WORKOUT.

It isn't a good idea to consume a large meal any closer than an hour and a half to two hours before a workout. If you're going to the gym straight from work, have a couple of pieces of fruit if you're hungry. Save your meal for after. If you eat a large meal just before working out, your digestive system will be busy working on digesting the food and you'll experience nausea when you begin lifting the weights.

DON'T EAT DIRECTLY AFTER A WORKOUT.

Wait at least an hour before you eat. Your blood is being circulated throughout your muscles. Let your system come to a restful state so you can digest the food properly. Chances are you won't feel like eating for an hour anyway. There's a natural turnoff to eating a heavy meal directly after working out.

PREPARE FOODS AHEAD OF TIME.

If your time is scarce, it's a good idea to cook up a pot of steamed broccoli, cauliflower, or other vegetable and have it ready when you come home from work. You may be famished, and instead of reaching for the peanut butter jar, you reach for the vegetables to tide you over while you're making dinner.

You can prepare various dishes ahead of time so that they only need to be heated up. If you're planning to eat lots of roasts and other meals that take an hour or two, why not invest in a microwave oven?

CARRY SNACK FOODS WITH YOU.

If you know you will be too busy to stop for a meal or a snack, why not carry some raw carrots, an apple, some raisins, a quartered cucumber, or some such food with you. A quick snack on the run can be just what you need to tide you over for an hour or two, until you can find the time to sit down and eat at your leisure. A snack would stop the slowing down of your metabolism and the overeating at the next meal.

EATING IF YOU GET HOME LATE IN THE EVENING

Suppose you go to the gym straight from work and stop off to do some chores. You may end up getting home about nine-thirty at night. You're planning to go to bed at about eleven. What should you do about food? Feel free to eat your regular meal. Even though it isn't ideal to eat a lot just before bed, eating up to 500 calories an hour or two before bed will not do great harm. We do it quite often and so do many in-shape women we know, although we all agree that this is not the ideal time to eat because there is not enough time to burn away the calories. If you do eat just before bed, try to stay active for about half an hour. Do the dishes, clean around the house, prepare your clothing for the next day—just stay active. If possible, a ten-minute walk would be great.

Remember, food is not an enemy. Dieting is a scientific process. There's nothing to fear. Enjoy food and enjoy working out. Life is too short to live in self-punishment, fear, and near starvation. There is a better way to go, and we're glad you're planning to try it.

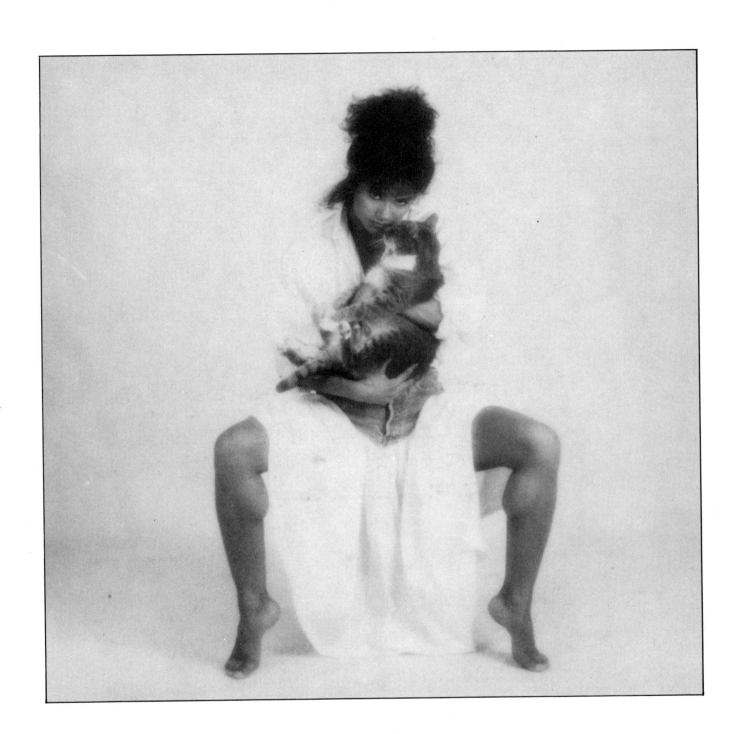

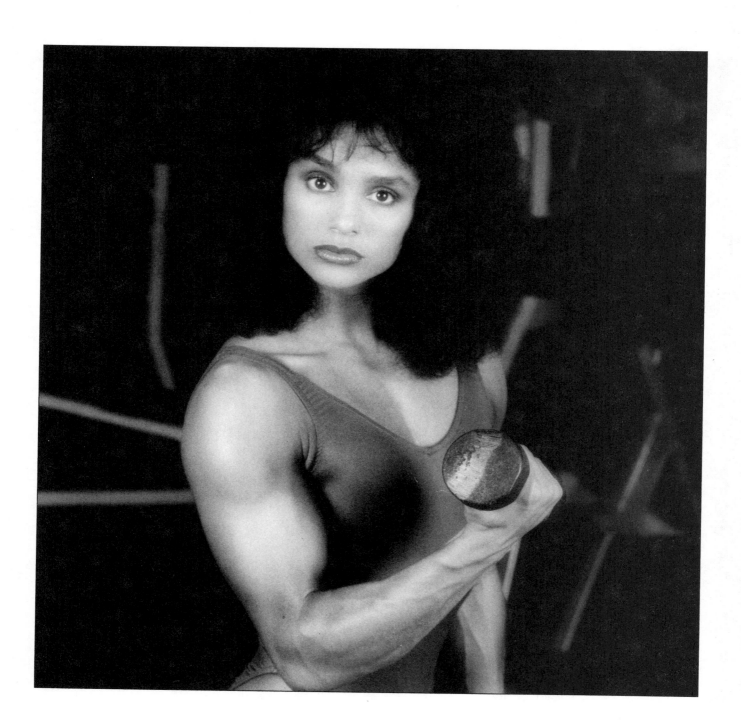

EIGHT

LIES, LIES, LIES: GLADYS AND JOYCE DISPENSE WITH THE SEVEN GREATEST MYTHS CONCERNING WOMEN AND WEIGHTS

"Won't I look like a man if I work out with weights?" "Doesn't it turn a man off to see or feel a woman who has muscles, even if she *doesn't* look like a man?" "Isn't it dangerous to work with weights—I mean, you could be seriously injured, right?" "Won't it all turn to flab once you stop?" "Isn't it boring to work with weights?" "Isn't it true that men and women have to do different exercises in order to get in shape?" "Won't I lose flexibility if I work out with weights?"

We have given fitness seminars around the country as well as abroad, and time and again these seven "worries" emerge. Women are afraid to train with weights because they have heard rumors. Well, it's time to realize that these rumors are passed down from one unschooled person to another until they develop into myths. It's time to break the seven myths with cold, hard facts that can be verified by doctors and other experts in the field of physical fitness.

MYTH #1. "YOU WILL LOOK LIKE A MAN IF YOU WORK WITH WEIGHTS."

This fear is based on pictures women have seen of female bodybuilders whose bodies do sometimes look more like men's than women's. We are personally acquainted with these women, and we happen to know that they spend a minimum of four hours a day in the gym and lift extremely heavy weights (with the assistance of "spotters"). In addition, some of these larger women have experimented with steroids and the male hormone testosterone, and have found to their dismay that there are undesirable side effects such as liver damage, difficulty in childbearing, and the development of male characteristics. For this reason, many of these women are now dropping the use of steroids, and we believe there will soon be a dramatic change in the appearance of female bodybuilding champions.

In any case, you can rest assured that you will not develop overly large muscles by following this program. It is carefully designed to create small, appealing muscles. There is no way you could possibly develop large, masculine-looking muscles by doing the exercises contained in this book, in the manner described.

MYTH # 2. IT TURNS A MAN OFF TO SEE OR FEEL A WOMAN WITH MUSCLES.

Not in our experience. We have found that quite the opposite is true. Men seem to love the look and feel of a firm, curvaceous female body. We have interviewed hundreds of women who are now in the kind of shape this program yields, and have asked them whether they were more appealing to men before or after they acquired muscles. Each of the women declared emphatically that they now feel more appealing, and that the difference in the positive male attention they now attract is quite surprising to them. It appears obvious that muscles on a woman, in the right proportion and in the right places, can only add to her sensuality.

MYTH #3. "IT'S DANGEROUS TO WORK WITH WEIGHTS."

Getting into shape with the use of weights is probably the safest method of achieving physical fitness. You control the weights, they do not control you. In any sport, you must be at the mercy of the element—the ball, the puck, the concrete, the opponent, and so on.

There is a natural warm-up provided with each exercise because of the pyramid system, so that injury even within the natural course of weight training is highly unlikely.

It is healthful rather than harmful to work with weights. As a matter of fact, it has been proven that osteoporosis, a bone condition that women become more susceptible to as they age, can be prevented and is often treated by working out with weights.

The condition of osteoporosis is caused by a decrease in bone mass. The coarse fibers in the bone are attenuated and the bone becomes hollow. With weight training, the coarse fibers in the bone become enlarged as a reaction to the stress placed on them by the weights. The result is an improved bone condition for women whose bones have already begun to lose mass, and a building up of mass against possible future hollowing for women whose bones have not yet begun to hollow. Weight training can do a lot more than any vitamin plan on the market; however, we do suggest proper eating as additional insurance against osteoporosis (see pp. 120–121).

Working with weights can also help to heal various injuries. For this reason, one of the major components of a physical therapy program is usually a carefully designed weight-training program. Such programs are recommended by doctors for use in healing back, knee, leg and other injuries. In short, working with weights the proper way is not harmful. It is therapeutic.

MYTH #4. "WON'T IT ALL TURN TO FLAB ONCE YOU STOP?"

No. Muscle is muscle and fat is fat, and never the twain shall meet. It is physically impossible for muscle to turn to fat. If you stop working out, your muscles will gradually shrink back to the size they were before you started working out. If you eat a lot and don't do something to burn up the calories, of course you will begin to get fat, but that has nothing whatsoever to do with the muscles you had that have begun to shrink. As a matter of fact, you are lucky to have at least had the muscles for a time, because those muscles will always "remember," and if you ever start working out again, it takes only one-fourth to one-third of the time you worked before to get back in shape. In other words, if you worked out for a year and stopped for a year, you might think you'd lost all of your muscles. But if you worked out again for three or four months, you would get back everything you lost. After that you would begin to progress even further. So every month you work out is a month of "muscle in the bank." In addition, it takes about as long as you trained to lose what you gained in muscle. For example, if you worked out for five years, it would take you five years to lose all the hard, pretty muscles you developed.

MYTH #5. "ISN'T IT BORING TO WORK WITH WEIGHTS?"

On the contrary. The hardest part is getting started. Once you pick up that first weight, the time flies by, and before you know it you're on your way out of the gym area. You wonder where the time went. Why? You are not doing the same monotonous, humdrum thing for the whole time. Instead you are kept interested by continuous change. You change your weights for each exercise and your exercises for each bodypart and eventually your bodypart for another bodypart—until suddenly you are finished. In addition to not being bored, you become totally absorbed in the workout, so much so that, in spite of yourself, you are forced to forget whatever problems you might have brought into the gym. Because the workout totally commands your attention, you feel as if you have taken a vacation from your problems. When you leave the gym, you are refreshed and invigorated. You have an improved mental attitude, and you feel as if you have done something exciting, not boring.

MYTH #6. "ISN'T IT TRUE THAT MEN AND WOMEN HAVE TO DO DIFFERENT EXERCISES IN ORDER TO GET IN SHAPE?"

No. As a matter of fact, men do exactly the same exercises as women. The only difference is, men do not have to do the buttocks exercise because nature has provided them with naturally narrow hips and less ample buttocks. The leg routine more than takes care of any stray buttocks problems a man would have. As far as the rest of the body goes, human anatomy is basically the same. A man and a woman can do the same exact exercise, but the man will naturally use a heavier weight because he is most likely stronger. In addition, a man's body will respond more dramatically to the weights and he will develop larger muscles. Why? A man has a naturally large supply of the male hormone testosterone, whereas a woman has a very tiny supply of this hormone.

MYTH #7. "WON'T I LOSE FLEXIBILITY IF I WORK WITH WEIGHTS?"

No. As a matter of fact you will become more flexible because you will have developed your overall body musculature in an even fashion. In addition, when you work with this program, you will find yourself doing a lot of "natural stretching." For example, after you do a squat, you will find yourself kicking out your legs and shaking them or bending over. This is your body's way of yawning—stretching itself out and elongating itself. When you do a lat pulldown, you may find yourself tempted to hang on the bar for a complete body stretch. All of this takes place because the body is coming into its own in flexibility and proportion. Finally, as you may have noticed, each exercise requires you to both flex, "squeeze together," and stretch for each repetition. Some of the most flexible people we know are bodybuilders, even the overly muscular ones. Haven't you ever noticed how the bulkiest of them can do difficult dance steps required for their posing routines at competitions?

We can't wait until you try this program for yourself, so that you can confirm that the above myths are ridiculous misconceptions, and so that you can help us to spread the word to other women that they, too, can begin to enjoy the exciting benefits that will immediately come to them from working out with weights—the right way.

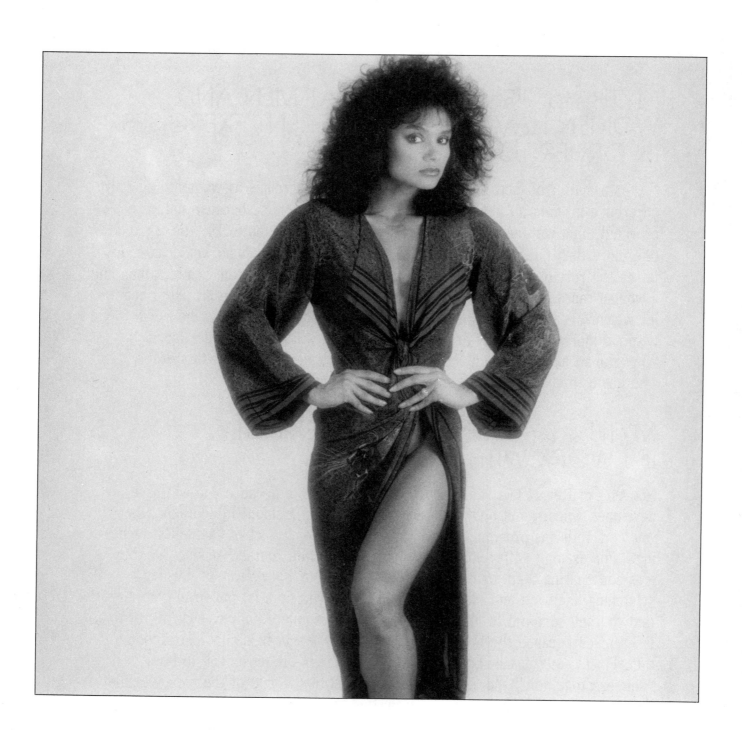

MORE THAN JUST A BEAUTIFUL BODY: POSITIVE EFFECTS IN OTHER AREAS OF LIFE

If the only thing you could get out of using this program was a beautiful body, you might be tempted to quit after a while. But you get a lot more than a reshaped body. You achieve a new mental attitude, better health, improved complexion and blood circulation, excellent posture, and increased stamina and agility in sports. Your general energy level increases. As an added bonus, you find that premenstrual syndrome is no longer an insoluble problem.

MENTAL ATTITUDE

Women have declared time and again that when they first begin their workout, they often feel depressed and reluctant to work out, yet by the end of the workout they have experienced a mood reversal. They become happy and cannot understand why. The reason is clear. The workout has caused the change.

The reason for the mood change can be explained in specific biological terms. Research has proven that the body produces natural morphine-like substances that work on the brain and spinal cord. These substances behave as opiates and are called endorphines. When a woman begins her workout, she may be depressed, but as she becomes involved in doing the exercises, her body relaxes. The blood begins to circulate. At the same time, her mind is forced to become involved with the specifics of the workout so that she cannot actively worry about her problems. While her mind and body are involved in the workout, she experiences positive thoughts that encourage the production of endorphines. When the endorphines are secreted by the brain, they behave as opiates. They block mental and physical discomfort. A feeling of well-being overtakes the person whose brain has secreted endorphines. It is evidently the secretion of these endorphines, resulting from the workout, that produces the "natural high" and relieves the individual from depression, worries, and negative mental attitudes.

RELIEF FROM PREMENSTRUAL SYNDROME

Since working out relaxes the body and produces a natural high, many women find that a good workout is the perfect antidote to premenstrual syndrome. It provides a welcome relief from the physical tension produced by the biological changes that take place in a woman's body before menstruation. Women have reported to us that they have been tempted to skip a workout when they felt weak and downcast because of the onset of menstruation; but they remember how great they always feel after a workout and force themselves to get to the gym. Afterward, these women report, they feel less cramping and are not as tense and irritable as they were when they entered the gym. They all declare enthusiastically that they are glad they overcame their initial reluctance to push themselves.

POSITIVE EFFECTS ON CIRCULATION AND SKIN TONE

One of the first things you'll notice after working out for a week or two is the improved tone and hue of your skin. Working with weights as prescribed in this book enables all of the major muscle groups to become stimulated directly. As you work your chest area, for example, the blood is forced to flow directly to that area in order to assist the muscle in tightening (flexing) and stretching so that it can lift and lower the weight. You work this way on your chest (and every other bodypart, for that matter) for about ten minutes. Since each body part is given direct attention for ten minutes and is afforded the treat of a fresh supply of blood for that time, the skin surrounding the area is stimulated and takes on a rosy coloring.

Even though you don't work on facial muscles, your complexion is also improved as a result of generally improved circulation. Many women report to us that people say they look younger since they have been working out and that their skin, which used to have an unhealthy, gray hue, now has a healthy, rosy tone.

IMPROVED POSTURE

Working out with weights develops the antigravity muscles. These are the muscles that determine your posture and your stance. Once you develop your muscles, your body no longer slumps downward, but rather stands tall. Your newly developed latissimus dorsi muscles (located in your back area) are strengthened so that your shoulders are held back rather than allowed to slouch forward. Your quadriceps (thigh) muscles become strong and defined so that instead of walking with a shuffle, you begin to walk with an athletic stride. Your trapezius muscles (located between your neck and shoulder area) are strengthened so that your head is held up strongly and is not thrust forward in an unattractive manner. All parts of your body are toned and tight and working together to give you perfect posture. Your bones are made stronger and denser so that they can support your body more efficiently.

IMPROVED STAMINA AND AGILITY IN SPORTS

Working out with weights increases your overall strength. It is generally recognized that if two people of equal talent and ability are competing against each other in a given sport, the stronger one will win the game. Getting stronger will definitely help your game.

Weight training also increases your flexibility. Because you are continually flexing and stretching each muscle as you work on it, you are increasing the ability of that muscle to respond to flexibility needs outside of the workout area—specifically, in your sport.

Tennis players experience greater strength in backhand shots, increased agility on the court, and improved stamina. There is more power available to racquetball, handball, and volleyball players.

Runners find that their running posture has improved, as well as their stamina. There are fewer aches and pains after a long, hard run because of the improved muscular coordination and strength. Bicycle riders are able to attain greater speeds because of increased quadriceps and hamstring strength, and experience less back pain because of highly developed back muscles and improved riding posture.

Dancers and participants in the martial arts find increased balance and coordination as well as strength.

Swimmers gain added power in the legs and arms, and are able to increase the distance previously achieved with a given stroke.

Today there are very few Olympic sports trainers who do not include weight training as a part of their regular conditioning program. Athletes use weights in order to meet the demands of their sport. For example, in gymnastics it is necessary for gymnasts to be able to lift their bodyweight for each movement. If gymnasts are weak, they can use weights as low as one-tenth of their bodyweight and work up to their full bodyweight. In time, they can even exceed their bodyweight, and make themselves stronger and stronger.

Step by step, little by little, weight training can give you a strong, flexible, healthy body that will result in the inevitable improvement of your ability in your sport.

A NEW YOU

You will achieve a new body and a new mind-set. As you work with weights you sweat out the old you—the tired, weak you—and breathe in the new energetic, strong you. You will stand taller, walk prouder, think more positively, and take on new challenges. The new you has an optimistic outlook on life. It says "I changed my body. I made myself strong. I can accomplish other things too." Everybody is looking for the fountain of youth. The fountain of youth is not found in water, it's found in weights—weights, used intelligently. Work with weights for six months and you'll feel and look ten years younger!

A SMALL PRICE TO PAY

Before you knew about this workout, you may have had a good excuse to procrastinate—to put off doing something about getting and staying in shape. You might have thought, quite understandably, "I can't afford to spend half of my time working out. I'm too busy." Now you know better. Just two workout sessions a week—that's all it takes. A small price to pay for a body that will never again hold you back from feeling wonderful about yourself—all the time.

BIBLIOGRAPHY

EXERCISE BOOKS FOR ADDITIONAL TRAINING

Portugues, Gladys, and Joyce L. Vedral, Ph.D. *Hard Bodies.* New York: Dell Publishing, 1986.

Vedral, Joyce L. *Now or Never.* New York: Warner Books, 1986.

NUTRITION BOOKS FOR ADDITIONAL INFORMATION

Hausman, Patricia. *The At-a-Glance Nutrition Counter.* New York: Ballantine Books, 1984.

Kirshbaum, John (ed.). *The Nutrition Almanac.* New York: McGraw-Hill, 1984.

Reynolds, Bill, and Joyce Vedral, Ph.D. *Supercut: Nutrition for the Ultimate Physique.* Chicago: Contemporary Books, 1985.

Tantum, Dr. Kermit R. *Shake the Salt Habit.* New York: Ballantine Books, 1981.

Vaughan, Dr. William. *Low Sugar Secrets for Your Diet.* New York: Warner Books, 1985.

STRETCHING

Friedberg, Ardy. *Reach for It.* New York: Simon & Schuster, 1985.

MAGAZINES

Muscle and Fitness, 21100 Erwin Street, Woodland Hills, CA 91367.

Shape, 21100 Erwin Street, Woodland Hills, CA 91367.

Female Bodybuilding, 475 Park Avenue South, NY, NY 10016.

INDEX

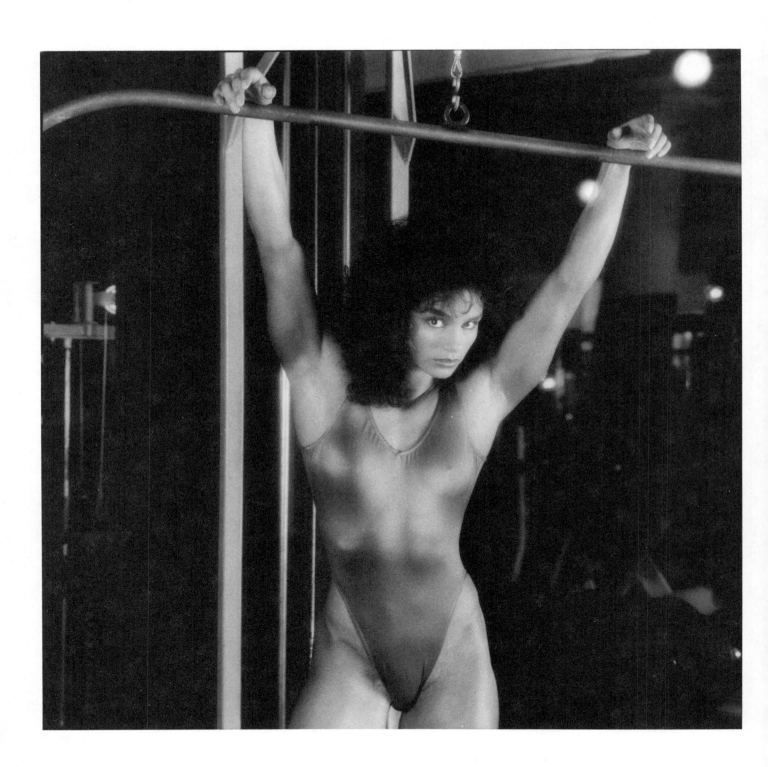